D1553758

Medical Practice Accounting & Finance

*A Practical Guide
for Physicians,
Dentists
and Other
Medical
Practitioners*

■ **Rose Marie L. Bukics**
Donald R. Chambers

A Healthcare 2000 Publication

 IRWIN
Professional Publishing®
Burr Ridge, Illinois
New York, New York

A **2000** *PUBLICATION*

This publication is designed to provide accurate and authoritative information in regard to the subject matter covered. It is sold with the understanding that the author and the publisher are not engaged in rendering legal, accounting, or other professional service.

ISBN 1-55738-630-7

Printed in the United States of America

BB

1 2 3 4 5 6 7 8 9 0

CB/BJS

To Joe, Karen, and Ali

As always, thanks for your patience!

RMB

Table of Contents

A Prescription for Better Financial Health

This book answers the questions asked most frequently by medical practitioners. A sample of those questions appears below.

1. Why does my medical practice show a profit but I don't have any cash?
   See Chapters 3 and 5

2. Should I lease or buy my office facilities and equipment?
   See Chapter 8

3. How can I increase my cash flow and control my operating costs?
   See Chapter 5

4. How can I protect my personal assets from the risks of business?
   See Chapter 2

5. How can I minimize my income tax?
   See Chapter 2

6. How much should I save in my pension plan?
   See Chapter 9

7. Where should I invest my pension money?
   See Chapter 9

8. Should I increase my office hours or add an additional office location?
   See Chapter 5

9. With only a few employees, how can I protect my business assets from unauthorized use or theft?
     See Chapter 7

10. What do I do with the financial information I receive from my accountant?
     See Chapters 1, 3, 4, 5, and 6

Acknowledgments

A special thanks to Doctors Donald B. Kopenhaver and Thomas S. Sauer, who spent a great deal of their personal and professional time assisting in the preparation of this book. Without their expert guidance, this book could not have been written.

The authors would also like to thank all of the medical professionals and others who willingly gave their time, energy, and ideas, as well as sharing their experiences and information. We are certain that their input helped us produce a book that makes a valuable contribution to the business education of medical professionals.

Anthony Abdalla, D.D.S.; Zoe Bilski, R.N.; Joseph D. Concetto, M.D.; Fabio Dorville, M.D.; Camille Eyvazzadeh, M.D.; Pamela Kametz, Office Manager; Wilbur Oakes, M.D.; Stanley Russin, M.D.; Steven Senft, M.D.; Ina Tuscano, Business Manager; Ivanna Vladkova.

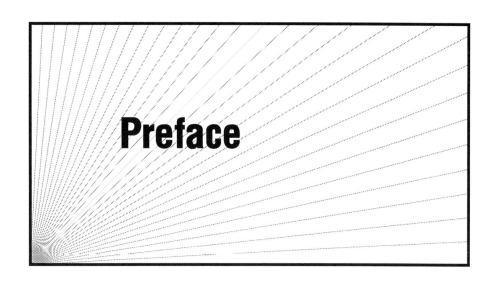

Preface

This book is written for physicians, dentists, and other health care professionals who have responsibility for, or an interest in, managing the business aspects of a health care practice. Health care professionals need to be much more than health care providers; they must also possess business, accounting, and financial skills. Yet, many physicians have virtually no background or training in such matters.

The book is intended to explain the fundamentals of accounting and finance, with specific application to a medical practice. Whether you are a solo health care provider or operate in a group practice, understanding the basic flow of accounting transactions and record-keeping is essential to comprehend the financial aspects of your business. In the book we will present financial statements and discuss them in terms of how monetary figures are reported and what impact they have on the daily operation of your practice. Only with an understanding of this information, can you, as a health care provider, make informed and intelligent decisions.

In addition, the book discusses general business practices that help insure an accurate and timely reporting of financial transactions. For example, one chapter is devoted to the need for, and development of, internal accounting controls used to protect your business assets. Additional consideration is given to lease versus buy options, which is helpful for those considering expansion of office facilities or the purchase of major equipment. The book concludes with a brief section on retirement and pension planning, an area which continues to grow in importance.

This book is designed to meet your need for financial information. It is designed both as a text with full explanations for most accounting and financial transactions, and as a valuable reference tool when questions arise. It may also supplement discussions with your accountant or banker, clarify transactions, or provide additional information.

We recommend that you read this book in sections. In certain cases, you may find that you need to read the material more than once to fully comprehend its meaning. But don't be alarmed if the material seems difficult. Just as you studied many years to become a physician, accounting and finance professionals spent many years mastering their specialty. Imagine your accountant trying to understand your procedures after reading a book once! Thus, frequent readings will facilitate your understanding of the material.

Given the current and expected changes in the health care environment, health care providers must be able to manage their medical practice as a business. After reading this book, you should have a better understanding of the accounting and finance procedures that form the foundation of business management. Mastering this information will allow you to make informed business decisions, which, in turn, will maximize the results of your medical practice.

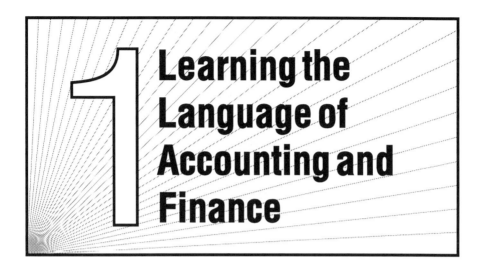

1 Learning the Language of Accounting and Finance

Dr. R. M. Lave winced as he counted the number of phone messages that he needed to return. There were seven messages—and he had only been gone an hour! But right now it was time to meet with his accountant and this time he vowed that it was going to be different. This time he would understand everything the accountant reported and would get control of his financial situation. . . .

How many times have you been involved in the situation described above? Physicians typically receive a copy of the accountant's report and meet with the accountant to review the results of the business. Yet, have you ever sat in the meeting vigorously nodding agreement, while the accountant provides volumes of information on your medical practice? When the accountant finishes the report and summarizes the highlights, it seems to make sense and you feel that you have a good grasp of the information. At the end of the meeting, you either file the report away or decide that you will review it again when you have more time.

When you subsequently examine the report, do you readily recall the information you discussed or do you decide that you didn't process as much as of the report as you initially thought? Does rereading the report leave you somewhat confused and/or do you have unanswered questions? Although you may feel frustrated and confused, you shouldn't be discouraged given the complexity of accounting and finance.

To overcome this obstacle, you need to focus initially on mastering the language of accounting and finance since it forms the foundation of all accounting and reporting of financial information for anyone in business. Understanding what the information means to your business is critical. Notice the words *your business!* In fact, medical practices today must be operated and managed in the same manner as any other business. Thus, having a thorough understanding of your financial results is imperative.

"Getting a handle" on the language of accounting and finance is the first step in helping you understand your business. It will also help you communicate with your accountant, bankers, and other professionals. Using an accountant's report as a guide, this chapter highlights the details of the financial information contained in an accountant's report and discusses the various types of accounting services available to you. The chapter also identifies the differences that you may find in your accountant's report. In reviewing the sample report, we will focus on key financial words and phrases and translate them into easily understood concepts. It might be helpful if you use a copy of your last accountant's report for reference.

This chapter will also introduce accounting and finance terms by examining both the accounting process and the accounting records that support your business activity. This is an area physicians typically either ignore or delegate to the trusted office manager. However, you *can* use the accounting process as an aid in managing the business aspects of your medical practice.

By the end of this chapter, you will be familiar with the terminology used by accountants and other business professionals. As a result, you should be able to

- Knowledgeably discuss the results of your business with your accountant and other professionals;
- Ask specific questions about your business results;
- Make intelligent and informed business decisions;
- Organize your accounting records to support the business aspects of your practice; and
- Follow a specific transaction from its inception to its reporting in the financial statements.

The Accountant's Report

An illustration of the standard accountant's report received by most physicians appears in Figure 1-1 for reference purposes. Take a minute to compare your report to the one produced below, noting any variations.

However, the first two paragraphs of the report should be virtually the same, regardless of the size of your practice, medical specialty, or the type of business organization. This is because standard reporting is dictated by the Statements on Standards established by the American Institute of Certified Public Accountants (AICPA), the accountant's professional organization.

The report starts with the standard two paragraphs noted below and we suggest the following treatment for these two paragraphs: (1) use this section of our book as a reference to help you understand what these paragraphs really mean, just once, then; (2) review your accountant's report each time it is received; (3) determine that these two paragraphs are the same; and (4) focus on the remaining information provided.

FIGURE 1-1
ILLUSTRATIVE COMPILATION REPORT

I/We have compiled the accompanying statements of assets, liabilities and stockholder's equity—modified cash basis of ABC Physicians Associates, as of December 31, 19xx and 19yy, and the related statements of revenues and expenses, stockholder's equity and cash flows—modified cash basis for the years then ended, and the accompanying supplementary disclosures, which is presented for supplementary analysis purposes, in accordance with standards established by the American Institute of Certified Public Accountants. These financial statements have been prepared on the cash basis of accounting, which is a comprehensive basis of accounting other than generally accepted accounting principles.

A compilation is limited to presenting, in the form of financial statements and supplementary disclosures, information that is the representation of management. I/We have not audited or reviewed the accompanying financial statements and supplementary disclosures and, accordingly, do not express an opinion or any form of assurance on them.

Thus, it is really important that you understand what these paragraphs mean, but since they usually repeat the same information each time, you don't need to spend time dwelling on their content.

We admit that these paragraphs are difficult reading, but once you understand what they mean, you only need to determine that your report contains the same paragraphs as the standard report. However, right now our job is to explain them carefully and completely so that you understand exactly what they say as well as their corresponding limitations.

Note that the first paragraph begins with "We have compiled . . . ." Although the definition and explanation of compilation services is explained in paragraph two, many people misunderstand the scope of these services. Thus, our discussion begins with an explanation of the services provided under a compilation.

What Are Compilation Services?

A compilation is the first level of accounting services provided by an accountant who is not an employee of your medical practice. Simply stated, this service takes the financial information produced by your medical practice accounting system and organizes the results into a standard reporting format.

It is important to note two items when discussing compilation services. The first is that the responsibility for the financial statement's numerical results remains with the medical practice. This is clearly stated in the compilation report in the first sentence of paragraph two: "A compilation is limited to presenting in the form of financial statements information that is the representation of management (owners)." Thus, the services provided by an accountant under a compilation in no way relieve you, the physician, of the ultimate responsibility for the financial information.

The second item of importance, related to the first, is the limit of the accountant's responsibility. Because they are only reporting information that is prepared by the medical practice accounting system, they do not accept responsibility for the specific content of the information. Rather, their responsibility is restricted to its presentation in a prescribed format.

The above discussion is not meant to imply that compilation services are of limited value to a medical practitioner. Often times, these services are provided in conjunction with other bookkeeping, accounting, consulting, or tax services. By performing compilation services, your accountant presents information in a standard format so that you can see your financial results in a clear, concise, and consistent manner. Thus, you can easily compare information from one period to another and analyze the significant changes. This focus is necessary for the business management of your medical practice.

Other Financial Statement Accounting Services Available

Although physicians typically use compilation services for their financial statements, it is also helpful to consider other levels of accounting services. Referring to the report, note that the last sentence of paragraph two explains that the financial statements and supplementary disclosures have not been *audited* or *reviewed*. An explanation and comparison of these terms to compilation services should be beneficial.

Review

A review is more in-depth than a compilation and includes the financial statement presentation previously described. However, a review also requires that your accountant make inquiries of your personnel and perform analytical procedures on the accounting information. Once again, the responsibility for the data remains with the physician.

A review also means that as a result of the additional procedures applied, your accountant concluded that the information in the financial statements did not require any significant changes. To illustrate, cash is reported in the financial statements in both a compilation and a review. However, in a review, your accountant would consider additional information related to the cash value reported. Examples of such information might be whether there are any restrictions on the availability of cash or whether the bank reconcilements have been performed.

Audit

An audit is the most in-depth accounting service available and provides assurance that the financial information is fairly presented. An audit does not mean that the accountant guarantees the accuracy of every number. Rather, the information appears to be reasonable, based on specific audit procedures applied.

Referring back to paragraph two of the illustrative report, notice that it specifically states that since an audit or review was not performed, no opinion or statement of assurance is given. This, once again, restates your responsibility for the numbers.

Financial Information in a Compilation Report

The first paragraph identifies that the compilation report accompanies the financial statements and typically, there are four statements (although not all practices have a statement of cash flows prepared). The first reference in this paragraph is to (1) the Statement of Assets, Liabilities and (shareholder's or stockholder's)Equity; (2) the basis on which it is prepared; and (3) the relevant time period.

The Statement of Assets, Liabilities and Equity

You can't understand the Statement of Assets, Liabilities and Equity if you don't understand what Assets, Liabilities and Equity are or what they mean to your practice. Assets can be thought of as the positive aspect of your business (e.g., cash, receivables, or equipment) since they are the financial resources owned and available for use in your practice.

Liabilities are the debts that the practice must repay, such as amounts owed to suppliers or the mortgage held by the bank on your building. Thus, liabilities represent a drain or negative impact on your finances.

Equity is comprised of either the ownership contributions made by the physician(s) or the amount of earnings that have been reinvested in the business over time. This accumulation of earnings in the business is appropriately called "retained earnings" and is a separate component in the equity structure of your business. (In cases of a sole practitioner or a partnership, the ownership interest and retained earnings are often not reported separately. Rather, they are combined and reported in your financial statements as a single capital or equity account.)

The Statement of Assets, Liabilities and Equity groups each of the elements together in a particular way. To illustrate, look at your statement and see how it identifies total assets available. Note that it also indicates total liabilities and equity and that the liabilities and equity combined equals the assets. This means that you can easily identify the source of the financing used to acquire your assets since all assets are acquired in one of three ways: (1) through a debt incurred by the practice; (2) by direct contribution of a physician's interest; or (3) by allowing the profits from the business to be reinvested in the practice (i.e., retained earnings). That is why assets will always equal liabilities plus equity. The Statement of Assets, Liabilities and Equity is the same as a balance sheet, which is the common title used for businesses other than medical practices.

The next reference to the Statement of Assets, Liabilities and Equity, is the basis on which it is prepared. The most common basis for medical practitioners is the modified cash basis or income tax basis of preparation. These methods are other than that used under "generally accepted accounting principles" (GAAP), which refers to the accrual method of accounting. An in-depth discussion of this basis of preparation will be presented in Chapter 3.

The third reference in paragraph one of the report is the dating of the Statement of Assets, Liabilities and Equity. This statement is the only one of the four financial statements that is dated at a specific point in time (i.e., as of the end of a month, quarter, or year). This means that the information on this statement is relevant only on that particular date. Chapter 4 has been devoted entirely to this financial statement.

Other Financial Statement Information

Now, reread the first paragraph of the compilation report and note that it also refers to (1) "the related Statement of Revenue and Expense" or "Revenue Collected and Expenses Paid" and (2) a Statement of Retained Earnings, or in some cases, a Statement of Shareholder's Equity. Some medical practices also prepare a Statement of Cash Flows.

An important and often overlooked word in the sentence describing the other financial statements is "related." Simply stated, the final number shown on the Statement of Revenues and Expenses (called net income) is the amount of revenue generated over the amount of expenses paid. This excess is then transferred to retained earnings and becomes new equity for the medical practice. This has the same effect as a physician making an additional cash investment in the practice.

Although this may appear to be complicated, it can be shown by examining the financial statements as a single unit, which we have illustrated in Figure 1-2. Note that net income from the Statement of Revenues and Expenses carries forward to increase the existing balance in the retained earnings account, which is shown on the Statement of Shareholder's Equity. The ending balance in retained earnings reported on that statement in turn carries forward to the shareholder's equity portion of the Statement of Assets, Liabilities and Equity.

The basis on which the financial statements are prepared, as well as the relevant time period covered for these related statements, are stated in the accountant's report. One item to note is that the Statement of Revenue and Expense, the statement of retained earnings or shareholder's equity, and the Statement of Cash Flows are always for a period of time. These statements are cumulative in nature for a month, quarter, or year in contrast to the Statement of Assets, Liabilities and Equity which is a "snapshot" of a specific point in time.

Additional information presented in the first paragraph of the accountant's report refers to supplementary information (i.e., any information other than the four financial statements) that is presented with the accountant's report. Included in this category are the notes to the financial statements. This is usually narrative information that provides additional details or supports the information presented in the financial statements.

The first paragraph in the accountant's report ends with reference to "standards" established by "the American Institute of Certified Public Accountants" (AICPA). The applicable standards to which they refer are prescribed by the AICPA, the accountant's professional organization, and these standards govern the services performed by accountants.

FIGURE 1-2
FINANCIAL STATEMENT INTERRELATIONSHIPS

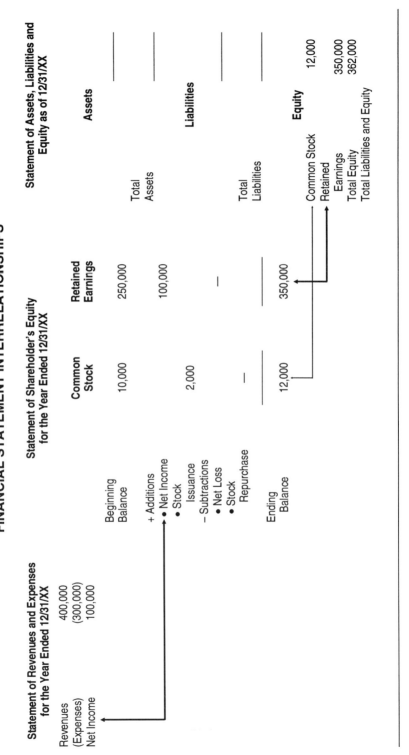

Statement of Revenues and Expenses for the Year Ended 12/31/XX

Revenues	400,000
(Expenses)	(300,000)
Net Income	100,000

Statement of Shareholder's Equity for the Year Ended 12/31/XX

	Common Stock	Retained Earnings
Beginning Balance	10,000	250,000
+ Additions		
• Net Income		100,000
• Stock Issuance	2,000	
– Subtractions		
• Net Loss		—
• Stock Repurchase	—	
Ending Balance	12,000	350,000

Statement of Assets, Liabilities and Equity as of 12/31/XX

Assets

Total Assets	____

Liabilities

Total Liabilities	____

Equity

Common Stock	12,000
Retained Earnings	350,000
Total Equity	362,000
Total Liabilities and Equity	

Report Modifications

When examining a copy of the report received from your accountant, you may see an additional paragraph after the two standard paragraphs discussed above. This paragraph is usually a statement concerning the omission of supplementary disclosures, such as the notes to the financial statements, or the omission of a Statement of Cash Flows. (If the statement of cash flows is in fact included as part of the financial statement package, reference to it would appear in the first paragraph, after the reference to the Statement of Retained Earnings or the Statement of Stockholder's Equity.)

The decision to omit this information rests with you, the physician. Omission of such data is common in the monthly, or even quarterly financial reporting. However, the disclosures are usually presented with year-end financial statements.

This third paragraph also states that if such information were included, it might affect the financial statement reader's conclusions concerning the entity's financial position, results of operations, or cash flows. This simply means that the reader's interpretation of the financial statements may be different if the additional information was presented.

This paragraph concludes with a statement as to the use of financial information that does not include such detail, and that should not be used by those that do not have access to the data. Thus, only participants in the practice who have direct knowledge of the additional information should use such data to make business decisions.

If you are the only reader of the financial statements and you are sole practitioner, such omissions are not normally a problem. However, these disclosures should not be omitted in the following cases: (1) where there are multiple physicians in the practice, or (2) if the financial statements will be used by those outside of the medical practice (e.g., a banker).

Now that we have thoroughly discussed the end product, the accountant's report, remember our earlier advice. Examine the report each time you receive it from your accountant to make sure it presents the standard information. Then, put it aside and focus on the numerical data contained in your financial statements. To help you with this issue, this chapter will now examine the daily activity of your medical practice from an accounting perspective and focus on the information flow that precedes the formal financial statement preparation. This will help you understand the accounting cycle that occurs continuously in your medical practice and we will illustrate how you can use the information as it is processed to manage your medical practice.

The Accounting Cycle

The accounting cycle begins with a single financial transaction and concludes with the formal summary of all transactions, presented in the form of your financial statements. The accounting cycle is exactly as its name implies, an ongoing, repetitious circle of accounting events that begins whenever a financial transaction occurs.

Financial transactions are those that affect any of your financial resources, debts, equity interest, revenues, or expenses. Payments received from clients, the purchase of supplies, the payment of employee salaries, or the purchase of a new piece of equipment are all examples of financial transactions that initiate the record-keeping process.

When the transaction occurs, it must be recorded in the accounting records. Since there is typically a high volume of transactions in your medical practice in a given time period, there must be a process that groups like transactions, so that you can see the net impact of all transactions on a specific account. For example, it is necessary to process the collection of cash receipts on a daily basis and the payments of cash as checks are processed. However, knowing each individual transaction is of limited value. As manager of a business, you need to know the net cash balance in the account at a specific point in time to determine the availability of cash for your current and future business needs. As a result, your accounting system must provide a process that frequently calculates the net impact of all transactions affecting the cash account.

Individual transactions are recorded as they happen. In contrast, the grouping process of like events occurs on a daily, weekly, or monthly basis, depending upon the size of your medical practice and your need for timely information. The greater the need for up-to-date information, the more frequently the process should occur. For example, if the lack of ready cash is a problem for your practice, good cash management becomes critical. Thus, cash receipts and disbursements should be promptly recorded.

Once the grouping process takes place, it is wise to summarize and verify the information before the next series of events occurs. This allows you to determine that the events recorded to date are properly represented and accounted for in the system. The cycle of recording information, grouping like transactions, and summarizing/verifying the information is illustrated in Figure 1-3. This cycle is actually repeated several times within a financial reporting period. The first is the result of your normal operating activities; the second, known as the adjusting phase, and the third, known as the closing process, occur whenever financial statements are prepared (i.e., monthly, quarterly, or annually).

If you understand the events described above and illustrated in Figure 1-3, you have mastered the accounting cycle. However, the accounting cycle has its own specific jargon, which we will now introduce in conjunction with the books of record used by an accounting system.

Accounting Records

There is always a tendency to think of an accounting system and its record-keeping function as a "necessary evil" used only to record the facts surrounding business activity. If you hold such a narrow view, it will, in fact, limit how you can use this process to manage your business. If you stop thinking about the accounting records as just part of a process in which you don't need to concern yourself, and consider these records as the source of vital information on your medical practice, they can be a tremendously useful management tool.

FIGURE 1-3
THE ACCOUNTING CYCLE

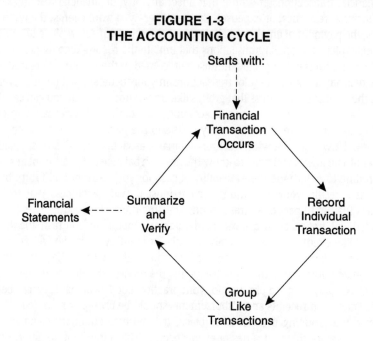

The recording of individual transactions occurs in specific accounting journals, depending upon the type of transaction involved. The journals most common to a medical practice are the cash receipts and cash disbursements journals. If your payroll process is handled internally, rather than contracted out to a payroll preparation company, you most likely will have a payroll journal. A general journal is also used when the accounting event cannot be recorded in any of the other mentioned journals.

Cash Receipts Journal

A cash receipts journal is exactly as its names implies, a document used to record your receipt of cash or checks. Every transaction is entered into two columns of the journal, one for the total cash received in a specific transaction, and another designating the source of the cash received. This is why accounting is referred to as a double entry bookkeeping system. To illustrate, the receipt of a check from a patient will be entered into the cash receipts journal in the total cash received column and in a second column designated as "professional fees" or "revenues earned."

Cash receipts journals also provide additional space for comments or notations as needed, such as a check number, date, and the individual or company from whom the cash was received. Whether the source of cash is from fees earned, payments on accounts receivable, money drawn against a line of credit, or rental revenue received from others who use your facilities, all receipts of cash must be entered into the accounting system through this single record.

A well-organized cash receipts journal provides the opportunity to separate and identify major sources of cash as they are received. Thus, you can organize the information in a manner that will support your decision-making needs. For example, it may be necessary or desirable to track fees earned for a particular physician, satellite office, or subspecialty within the group practice. Perhaps you may need to track revenues earned by a satellite office located in a different municipality and subject to a separate taxing authority. Or an allergist may find it useful to determine the fees earned from allergy injections as a separate component of revenues generated.

If you determine in advance the type of information you want or need and how often it is needed, you can easily design the record-keeping process, beginning with the initial recording of a transaction, to accomplish this goal. It is wise to use this flexibility to acquire relevant information easily and in a timely manner.

Cash Disbursements Journals

Cash disbursements journals are organized in a manner similar to that of the cash receipts journal where one column is used for the total cash outlay and the other columns classify the type of expenditure. These additional columns are usually titled for the most common expenses caused by cash disbursements, such as medical supplies, rent, utilities, office supplies, salaries (unless a separate payroll journal is maintained), insurance, and so on. In addition, information such as the check payee, number, date, and other explanations, will also be noted.

Other Journals

If your practice maintains a payroll journal, disbursements to your employees will be recorded in this journal. (However, the payment of salaries can also be handled by the regular cash disbursements journal as noted above.)

Recording accounting events that do not impact cash receipts or cash disbursements, such as the depreciation of equipment, will usually be shown in the general journal. Depending on the size of your medical practice and the sophistication of your accounting system, your practice may also use a purchases journal.

Information should be recorded in the appropriate accounting journal as each individual transaction occurs. At a predetermined, fixed interval (e.g. daily, weekly, or monthly) the total for each column is calculated. These amounts then form the basis for the next step in the recording process, known as the journal entry.

Journal Entries

Journal entries are used to organize initial accounting data for entry into the next accounting record, the general ledger. A journal entry is comprised of debits and credits, a date, and an explanation. It is not necessary to understand what a debit and credit mean, they are merely accounting terms for increases and decreases in an account.

However, not all debits are increases, nor are all credits decreases. Rather, debits to asset and expense accounts are increases, with credits as decreases. For liability, equity, and revenue accounts, debits are decreases and credits are increases. If you think of assets as the opposite of liabilities and equity, and revenues as the opposite of expenses, the fact that the debits and credits are in the opposite direction should also make sense.

The Posting Process and the General Ledger

Once financial transactions have been recorded in their respective journals, the grouping of like transactions described earlier, takes place. This process, called *posting*, uses the debits and credits recorded by the journal entries and transfers them to the master accounting record, known as the general ledger. This ledger organizes the information by specific accounts such as cash, equipment, or utility expense. After all the journal entries are posted in the general ledger, a balance for each account is calculated and that balance is reported in your financial statements.

Each type of general ledger account, whether asset, liability, equity, revenue, or expense, has its own respective section of the general ledger, coded by the use of account numbers. For example, assets may be assigned account numbers 1000 through 1999, liabilities are accounts 2000 through 2999, etc. There is no limit or restriction as to how a general ledger is organized. You can tailor it to meet the needs of your medical practice. Smaller medical practices with fewer accounts may have a two-digit general ledger account sequence, while larger practices may use a three- or four-digit sequence. Although the posting process is the same for any company, how you structure the general ledger for recording your medical practice results is determined by your individual information needs.

To illustrate the accounting cycle thus far, assume that your practice received payments from 25 patients for services rendered on a given day. Each individual payment has been entered into the cash receipts journal as it is received and the cash receipts for the day total $1250. The journal entry that results is an increase (or debit) to the cash account and an increase (or credit) to your professional fees earned account. The posting of this transaction increases the existing balance in each of these accounts to reflect that you now have more cash than you previously did because additional fees have been earned.

Preparation of the Trial Balance

The next step of the accounting cycle is critical. The summarization/verification phase, known as preparation of a trial balance, lists every general ledger account and their respective debit or credit balances. The point of this exercise is to determine that the sum of all debit accounts equals the sum of all credit accounts. If this in fact occurs, it means that your accounting records are in balance. If not, it is necessary to go back to the previous phases of the accounting cycle and determine if an error was made in the journal entry recording or in the posting to the general ledger.

Balancing the accounting records at this phase makes it easier to find and correct errors prior to beginning the accounting cycle again. Assuming no additional transactions, the financial statement preparation described earlier in the chapter, can be completed after the preparation of the trial balance. It may be helpful now to examine Figure 1-4, which looks like Figure 1-3, but is revised to show the description of the accounting cycle in conjunction with the specific accounting records used.

The Adjusting Entries

The cycle of recording journal entries, posting to the general ledger, and preparing a trial balance, actually occurs at three distinct times. The first records the ongoing, daily operating activities described earlier.

However, there are additional entries, known as adjusting journal entries, that must be periodically recorded in the general journal. Adjusting journal entries insure that all financial transactions impacting the business in a given time period are recorded. For those larger medical practices who routinely employ an accountant on staff, these journal entries are part of their normal job responsibilities. However, in smaller medical practices, these adjustments are normally part of the services provided by an outside accountant.

The most common adjusting journal entries record depreciation of equipment, and reflect adjustments to accounting information previously recorded. To illustrate, assume your practice purchased a large amount of medical supplies and recorded the purchase as prepaid medical supplies because the supplies were to be used over an extended time period. Since prepaid supplies are an asset, the balance would be shown on the Statement of Assets, Liabilities and Equity as a financial resource available for use. However, it is necessary to determine the amount of supplies used and to record this amount as an expense in the time period corresponding to their use. Thus, the adjusting journal entry would decrease the prepaid supplies account and increase the operating expense account for the period.

Once the adjusting journal entry is recorded in the general journal, it is posted to the general ledger and a new trial balance is prepared. This will indicate whether the accounting records remain in balance. At this point, the final phase, known as the closing process, can begin.

The Closing Entries

This cycle occurs for the third time when the books are "closed." This closing process accomplishes two things. First, since revenue and expense data are always reported for a period of time, it is necessary to zero out the revenue and expense accounts after each accounting period. This prepares the accounts to receive accounting information in a future period without commingling data from earlier accounting periods.

The closing process also calculates your actual earnings for the current period and transfers the balance to the equity accounts. The impact of this process on the financial statements was shown in Figure 1-2. However, the accounting records which support your financial statement information, must also reflect the closing transactions. Thus, closing journal entries are recorded, posted to the general ledger, and a trial balance is prepared.

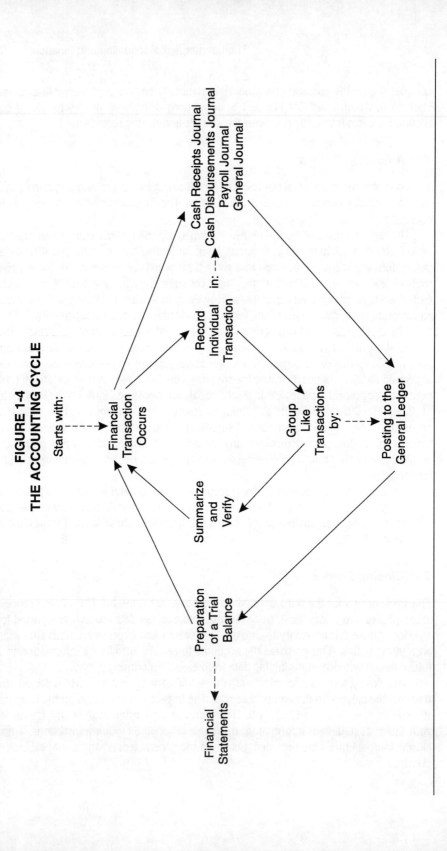

FIGURE 1-4
THE ACCOUNTING CYCLE

Starts with:

Financial Transaction Occurs

Record Individual Transaction

Cash Receipts Journal
Cash Disbursements Journal
Payroll Journal
General Journal

Group Like Transactions by:

Posting to the General Ledger

Summarize and Verify

Preparation of a Trial Balance

Financial Statements

To summarize, the accounting cycle is a process of recording individual transactions, grouping them by like account, and preparing a trial balance to determine that the information, as processed, balances. This process actually occurs at three distinct time intervals: (1) during normal operating activities; (2) in adjusting transactions; and (3) in the closing process. Whether your accounting records are manually prepared or computer generated, the process is identical.

Other Accounting Records

Another commonly used accounting record is the accounts receivable subledger. This record contains a complete listing of all patients and the balances owed to the medical practice for services you previously provided. The amount may be due from either the patient or the insurance company. Information is entered into this accounting record whenever a transaction affects an individual patient account. Thus, receipt of payment from a patient is reflected in the cash receipts journal as described earlier but must also be recorded as a reduction in the patient balance in their individual ledger account.

Physician's Checklist

As a summary of the chapter, ask yourself the following questions with respect to your medical practice. If you can answer "yes" to these questions, you have a good understanding of the language of accounting and finance.

_____ 1. Do you know who has responsibility for the financial statement data?

_____ 2. Do you understand how net income transfers from the Statement of Revenues and Expense to the Statement of Assets, Liabilities and Equity?

_____ 3. Are your cash receipts and disbursements journals organized to provide timely and relevant financial information?

_____ 4. Do you understand the compilation report received from you accountant?

_____ 5.   Can you follow a financial transaction through the accounting records—from its initial journal recording, to the general ledger and trial balance, and ultimately, to the financial statements?

Understanding the financial terminology sets the stage for the remainder of this book. The accounting and financial process and record-keeping tools described in this chapter are the same regardless of the size of your medical practice, daily operating activity, medical specialty, or form of business organization.

However, there are distinct tax and legal differences in the various forms of business organization. Most physicians are unaware of what it means to have the practice organized and operating as a sole proprietorship, partnership, "S" corporation, or a professional corporation (PC). Chapter 2 will highlight the important points of interest for each of these forms of organization. If you are knowledgeable about this information, you can skip Chapter 2 and proceed to the discussion of financial statement fundamentals in Chapter 3.

Questions and Answers

1. Who has responsibility for the financial statement information?

You, as the owner of a medical practice, have responsibility for the financial statement information. Although the financial statements may be prepared by an accountant not employed by the practice, they remain your responsibility.

2. How valuable are the reports I receive from my accountant?

The reports you receive from your accountant are as valuable as you make them. They summarize financial information and report on past results. Therefore, you can use this information to judge your effectiveness relative to another time period. The accountant's report also allows you to see how a particular financial event fits into the total financial picture of your medical practice. The information provided by your accountant should be reviewed by you on a monthly basis.

3. What should I do with the accounting information that I receive from my accountant?

The information that you receive from your accountant should be reviewed by you at least monthly, with additional time and attention at quarter and year end.

In addition, you should consider "translating" this information into another, more usable format, such as common-sizing financial statements. This means restating the financial statements using one financial statement element as the common denominator. You can also prepare a trend analysis, which focuses on a particular element over the last three to five years. Third, you can prepare financial ratio information, which relates specific financial statement information in a numerator/denominator format. See Chapter 3 for specific details.

4. My accountant's report refers to the "basis" of my financial accounting information. What are the bases of accounting information and what do they mean?

Your financial statements can be prepared on a cash or accrual basis of accounting. You may also see your accountant's report refer to a modified cash basis or an income tax basis of preparation.

A cash basis records financial transactions only when cash is received or paid. An accrual basis report means that the revenue or income was recorded when it was earned, and the expenses were recorded while they were incurred regardless of whether cash was involved.

A modified cash basis and income tax basis are essentially the same. This basis means that transactions were initially recorded when cash was received or paid, but additional noncash transactions, such as depreciation expense, are also recorded as adjustments to cash basis information.

5. **My financial statements are accompanied by an accountant's report known as a compilation. What does this mean?**

A compilation is the first level of services provided by an accountant who is not an employee of the medical practice. A compilation uses the financial information produced by the medical practice's accounting system and organizes it into a standard reporting format.

6. **What is the accounting cycle and why is it important?**

The accounting cycle describes the length of time required to record, process, and summarize your financial transactions. It begins with a single financial event and ends with a summary of financial results. The accounting cycle is important because it establishes a standard reporting period for summarizing your financial results.

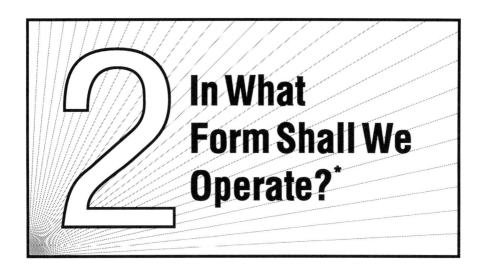

2 In What Form Shall We Operate?*

Dr. Lave is confused! He just returned from a conference where he saw many of his colleagues from medical school. One night at dinner Dr. Smith, a pediatrician, asked Dr. Lave how his practice was organized. Dr. Lave operates his practice as a Professional Corporation, generally known as a PC. Dr. Smith said his business was organized as a partnership and wanted to know why Dr. Lave was organized as a PC.

This is where Dr. Lave's confusion began. Although his accountant and attorney gave reasons when they recommended that he start his practice as a PC, now he cannot recall the specific advantages or disadvantages of that form of organization. In addition, he is beginning to wonder if the tax and legal considerations have changed to make other forms of business organizations more beneficial to a physician. As a result, he decides to schedule a meeting with his attorney, and asks his CPA to be present.

At the meeting, the attorney tells Dr. Lave that he talked with the CPA prior to the meeting and is glad that the accountant is present today. The lawyer informs Dr. Lave that good representation means having a good working relationship with everyone on the financial team, especially the accountant. This is necessary because of the many items that need coordination between the attorney and accountant, and sharing information produces a better result.

Dr. Lave tells his lawyer that he wants to know why he is organized as a PC and what benefits he has with that form of organization. The lawyer responds that to understand why you are practicing as a PC, it is helpful to discuss and understand the various alternative forms of business organizations in which you might operate a medical practice.

This chapter was written by Stanley E. Stettz, President, Teel, Stettz, Shimer & DiGiacomo, Ltd., Easton, Pennsylvania. B.S. in Accounting, Magna Cum Laude 1961, University of Scranton. J.D. 1964 Dickinson School of Law, Woolsack Society, Assistant Editor of the Law Review. Lafayette College Instructor in Economics – Business Law.

Let's discuss them as though you have no previous knowledge about the operation of a practice in any type of business form. Throughout this discussion, we will focus on protecting your personal assets from your business risks as well as the effect of taxation on the various forms of business organizations.

As we review the various business organizations, we will highlight the amount of personal protection you would have if you were to use each of the forms of organization. Stated differently, what business form will best protect you from losing your personal assets and yet provide favorable tax treatment? As you know, today it seems as though everyone is looking for a reason to sue—justified or unjustified. In addition everyone needs to consider tax consequences.

This chapter will address Dr. Lave's concerns. Specifically, it will answer the following questions:

- What forms of business organization are available to a medical practitioner?
- What are the legal effects of each form?
- What are the tax effects of each form?
- What are the advantages and disadvantages of each form of organization?

However, before we begin our discussion, you must consider the fact that regardless of the business organization, the following legal principles always apply:

1. **Every person is personally and financially responsible for his or her actions.**

2. **If a person is acting as your agent, you may also be responsible for the actions of that person.**

Consider the following example. During the course of surgery you negligently cause harm to your patient. As a result, you are personally responsible. If you have a physician assistant during the surgery and the assistant negligently causes harm, the assistant is personally responsible. However, you are also personally liable for the assistant's acts because he or she is considered as acting on your behalf. This is known as the Law of Agency. The above principles apply regardless of the form of business organization.

The next three sections of this chapter introduce the various forms of business organizations and discuss the legal and tax aspects. In order to communicate with your attorney and accountant, it is usually useful to have a general understanding of each form of business organization.

Forms of Business Organizations

Although there are many forms of business organizations, our discussion will deal only with those considered as the traditional forms in which medical practices are conducted. Therefore, our discussion will focus on sole proprietorships, general partnerships, "S" corporations, professional corporations, and the new limited liability companies. We will also discuss limited partnerships because physicians are often approached to personally invest in limited partnerships and they logically follow a discussion of partnership.

This section overviews the relevant forms of business organization. The next two sections will detail the legal and tax aspects.

Sole Proprietorship

When you conduct business as a sole proprietor, there is no separate business organization. You simply use your personal assets for business purposes. Therefore, a sole proprietor operates a business as an individual. There is no distinct legal entity.

General Partnership

A general partnership brings together two or more persons who seek to run a business for profit as co-owners. The term *persons* is intentionally used rather than the term *people*. For general partnership purposes, the term *persons* is broader than *people* and includes partnerships, corporations, and other types of legal associations. Thus, for example, two corporations can form a general partnership.

A partnership may be created by an oral or written agreement. There is no law governing the creation of a partnership. It is not a separate entity, but is simply a grouping together of persons.

Limited Partnership

Although medical practices are not organized as limited partnerships, we include a brief discussion of this form of organization because it is one type of investment that you may be asked to undertake in other types of business activity. Its formation is completely different from a general partnership in that there are strict filing and legal procedures which must be followed. The formation of a limited partnership can give the limited partners some protection from personal liability for the acts of other investors.

Corporations

In discussing corporations, you should be aware that there are various types of corporations. There are public corporations, not-for-profit corporations, and private corporations, among others. We will consider only "S" corporations and professional corporations in our discussion because they are the type of corporations used by medical practitioners.

Now let's compare domestic and foreign corporations. With the advent of HMOs and other managed care organizations, you may be part of a corporation classified as a domestic corporation in one state but simultaneously classified as a foreign corporation in another state. An HMO created under the laws of the state in which it does business is a domestic corporation. If it also does business in another state, there it would be classified as a foreign corporation. When a group of professionals, such as physicians, attorneys, or engineers, come together to operate their business in the corporate form, they do so as a professional corporation.

Limited Liability Company

A Limited Liability Company (LLC) is a relatively new form of business organization which has been sanctioned by the vast majority of states. An LLC combines the advantages of a partnership, such as taxation, with the advantages of a corporation, such as asset protection.

Legal Aspects of the Forms of Business Organizations

Having introduced and summarized the forms of business organizations that we will discuss, we turn to the legal aspects. Specifically, this section focuses on issues of liability.

Sole Proprietorship

Remember, a sole proprietorship is not a distinct legal entity. Therefore, the legal aspects of a sole proprietorship are those that define it as a person using personal assets to engage in a business. All of the liability that is imposed on your medical practice is imposed on you as an individual.

General Partnership

As we have noted, a partnership is not a separate legal entity different from the partners. What then is the liability of each member of the partnership? While there are various types of liability, we focus on negligent conduct (malpractice) and breach of contract. In the general partnership, all of the members may be sued in one action or separate actions may be lodged against each member. To illustrate, consider the following example:

> ABC Partnership consists of three physicians: Dr. Adams, Dr. Brown, and Dr. Care. The partnership has net assets after paying all liabilities of $200,000. Each doctor shares equally in profits and losses. Dr. Adams has personal assets of $1,000,000. Dr. Brown has personal assets of $400,000. Dr. Care has personal assets of $90,000. Dr. Care commits malpractice and a jury awards the patient $900,000.

Remember that the general partnership is not a separate legal entity, but simply a grouping of two or more persons to carry on business as co-owners. Since they are co-owners and partners, they are each responsible for the actions of one another. Partners receive the benefits of the business and must bear the losses of the business. It does not matter that they share profits and losses equally or unequally. Therefore, when Dr. Care causes a malpractice liability of $900,000, Dr. Care as well as Dr. Adams and Dr. Brown are responsible for this payment.

The patient now seeks to collect the $900,000 verdict. Dr. Care thinks that the partners have medical malpractice insurance. But what if the insurance had inadvertently lapsed? What if the insurance company is in financial trouble?

Further, what if the verdict was for punitive damages? Dr. Care says don't worry. Our insurance coverage takes care of all liability for which we are responsible. Wrong! Medical malpractice insurance does not provide coverage for punitive damages.

What if the verdict was in excess of the amount of insurance maintained by the partnership? Dr. Care would be responsible for the excess not covered by the insurance. However, not only is Dr. Care exposed, but also Dr. Adams, Dr. Brown, and the ABC Partnership.

If there is inadequate or no insurance, the patient decides from whom the verdict will be collected. The patient will select the course of least resistance in the collection. The partnership has assets of $200,000. Dr. Care only has assets of $90,000. The payment of the partnership's $200,000 and Dr. Care's $90,000 to the patient would still be insufficient to satisfy the verdict of $900,000.

What about Dr. Adams and Dr. Brown? They have a combined personal worth of $1,400,000. The patient will probably determine that the easiest way to collect the $900,000 would be to enforce the entire verdict against Dr. Adams and Dr. Brown since they have substantial assets. Dr. Adams and Dr. Brown then become responsible for payment, even though Dr. Care was negligent.

However, Dr. Care committed the wrongful act and is obligated to reimburse Dr. Adams and Dr. Brown for any money damages paid to the patient. In reality, Dr. Care has few assets, therefore, reimbursement would be unlikely. Thus, each partner's personal assets are at risk in a general partnership.

Limited Partnership

Although medical practices are not organized as limited partnerships, your investment in a real estate venture may well be. Thus, you should be aware of the aspects of this form of organization.

A limited partnership is formed by complying with a state law and is often used as an investment vehicle because it protects your personal assets. There must be at least one general partner and there can be one or more limited partners. The general partner is responsible for the acts of the partnership while the limited partners are protected from the acts of the other partners.

The limited partnership differs from a general partnership in several fundamental ways:

1. A general partnership may be formed by agreement and no statutory authority is necessary. However, a state statute which provides for the formation of limited partnerships must exist.

2. General partnerships have no filing requirements and may be formed by written or oral agreement. However, the limited partnership must comply with the requirements of the statute, including the appropriate filings in the office of the Secretary of State.

3. In a general partnership, each partner bears the risk of unlimited liability. In contrast, the liability of a limited partner is typically limited to the amount of money he or she has contributed, or agreed to contribute, to the partnership.

A limited partner cannot participate in the management of the partnership because that kind of activity could expose their personal assets to liability on behalf of the limited partnership. Basically, a limited partner should be a passive, rather than active, investor in a limited partnership.

Corporations

Now, we will deal with the concept of a corporation and how it does, and does not, protect you from personal liability. For discussion purposes here, assume that we are discussing a professional corporation.

To begin, consider the following question. If you own Union Carbide stock, a corporation whose shares are publicly traded on the New York Stock Exchange, should you be concerned about personal liability for the actions of Union Carbide? The answer is no. Would you be concerned if the stock you own was not traded on the New York Stock Exchange, or any other exchange? The answer is no. Would your concern change with the number of shareholders, whether it be 1, 2, 10, or 100,000 shareholders? As long as the shareholder's participation is limited to his or her role as an investor, the answer is no. Every shareholder, regardless of whether the corporate stock is publicly traded or privately held, has the same rights and privileges as every other shareholder, whether it is Union Carbide or John Jones, Inc., a one shareholder corporation.

The reaction that an individual shareholder should not be personally liable for a publicly traded corporation's liabilities is so common that it is almost a universal given. However, when we talk about small corporations, 1, 2, or 10 shareholders, people tend to question their status as shareholders and their potential personal liability.

The Corporation as an Entity

Let's consider the primary characteristics of the corporation. A corporation is a distinct legal entity—a creature of a statute. To bring a corporation into existence, Articles of Incorporation must be filed with the Secretary of State. It is a legal entity, with separate rights and separate liabilities.

A corporation is separate and distinct from its owners. The debts of the corporation are not the debts of the owners, directors, or officers. The existence of the corporate entity absolves the owners from the liabilities of the corporation. This separation of liability is generally known as the "limited liability concept" and it is the **main advantage** of the corporation. If the corporation fails, the only loss that the owner suffers is the amount of their investment in the shares of stock.

The stock of the corporation represents the owner's prorata ownership in the corporation. If you own 1,000 shares of your medical practice corporation, in which 5,000 shares are issued and outstanding, you own 20 percent of the practice.

Management

The day-to-day operations of a corporation are delegated to the officers of the corporation, who are elected by the Board of Directors. The officers, in turn, hire employees to perform the required tasks of the corporation, with the officers exercising direct managerial control. This organizational flow exists in every corporation regardless of whether there are 1,000 shareholders or 1 shareholder, or if its assets are $10,000 or $1,000,000. In a PC, the shareholders will usually act as the directors and officers.

Limited Liability

Since a corporation is separate and distinct from its owners, it creates a wall or veil between it and its owners, thereby insulating the owners' personal assets from any corporate liability. When a corporation has insufficient assets, or is used for illegal purposes, or not treated as a separate entity by its owners, creditors may try to pierce the veil or wall to reach the shareholders' personal assets. To avoid this consequence, the **formalities** of the corporate form **should be followed**. Make sure that minutes of the Board of Directors and Shareholders meetings are maintained. Sign documents in your corporate capacity, not as an individual.

The corporation can protect you as an individual by limiting your liability to your investment in the corporation. Recall our original principles of law: Every person is personally and financially responsible for their actions, and that of their agents.

It is important to note that the limited liability discussed above refers to protection allowed to investors. If a shareholder is actively involved in the management of the firm, then the shareholder can be legally exposed to liability resulting from that role.

Now that you know the basic information about the legalities of each form of organization, let's reexamine Dr. Lave's original question: Why is my practice organized as a professional corporation?

From a liability perspective, is it more advantageous for a group of doctors to operate as a professional corporation or as a general partnership? The answer should now be clear. In a general partnership, Dr. Adams cannot escape the potential liability for the malpractice of Dr. Care. In a professional corporation, Dr. Adams's personal assets are not exposed because of a judgment against Dr. Care. Therefore, only the assets of the corporation and the personal assets of Dr. Care are at risk.

This is a major reason why professionals form a professional corporation and practice in that form. Each physician becomes an employee of the corporation and as long as the physician does not personally, or through an agent, commit a wrongful act, the physician or other professional has no personal liability.

Limited Liability Company

Legislation has been adopted by many states, allowing the formation of a new type of business entity, the Limited Liability Company (LLC). Most of the legislation has been enacted within the last two years and at the time of this writing there are only three states, Hawaii, Massachusetts, and Vermont, without such legislation. In dealing with an LLC, each state's statute must be reviewed to insure proper formation of the LLC to obtain full use of its benefits.

Formation

The LLC is generally formed by filing Articles of Organization with the Secretary of State in the state in which it is formed. The Articles of Organization contain certain basic information, such as the principal place of business, the purpose for which it is formed, and the names and addresses of the initial management. This is similar to the content required in the Articles of Incorporation. In addition, it must contain a date which is the latest date in which the LLC must dissolve.

The LLC can be formed by two or more owner participants, who are generally called *members*. The LLC has the limited liability aspect of a corporation. It also limits a member's liability to their investment in the LLC unless the member, or their agent, commits a wrongful act of omission or commission. The LLC permits any type of entity to be a member.

Members

In the LLC statutes, members are not liable for the debts or claims against the LLC in the same way that shareholders do not have responsibility for the debts or claims of their corporations. The members of the LLC can be involved in the management of the business without subjecting themselves to personal liability, unlike the limited partnership.

The LLC may have different classes of members. For example, voting or nonvoting members, different distributions as they relate to items of income and loss, or different allocations of items of income or expenses for income tax purposes.

Management

The operation and management of the LLC is set forth in an operating agreement. This agreement typically addresses managerial responsibilities of the members, voting rights, distributions and other allocations, the rights of withdrawing members, and any restrictions on the transfer of interests. Unlike the Articles of Organization, the operating agreement need not be filed with the Secretary of State, and therefore, is not a public document.

Tax Aspects of Business Organizations

The next major issue in selecting a business organization is taxes. The key issue in each case is whether the business entity itself is taxed or whether the profits from the business entity flow immediately and directly to the personal tax returns of the owners.

Sole Proprietorship

The sole proprietorship is the equivalent of doing business as an individual, and accordingly, it has no impact on an individual's tax result. The same tax result that you now have as an individual you will have as a sole proprietor. Your business activity will be reported on Schedule C and filed with your 1040 income tax return.

General Partnership

A partnership is not required to pay federal income tax, but must file an information return giving the name of each partner and the amount of each partner's income or loss from the partnership. To understand a partnership for tax purposes, think of it as a pipe or conduit through which all of the revenues and expenses flow directly to the individual partners. Therefore, the operating results of the partnership are again reported by the individual on their income tax return, and as a sole proprietorship, it does not alter an individual's tax result.

Limited Partnership

For income tax purposes, the limited partnership is treated as a general partnership. Therefore, it is a conduit for the profits and losses to be distributed to the general and limited partners. This results in the inclusion of the profits or losses on each individual partner's personal income tax return. This form of business organization does not impact on an individual's tax result.

Corporations

For income tax purposes, medical practices organized as a Professional Corporation (PC) can be a "C" corporation or an "S" corporation, each having separate income tax results.

"S" Corporation

Congress determined that the form of business organization in which an individual chooses to operate his or her business should not be dictated by income tax rates. Accordingly, the Internal Revenue Code permits a tax election by the shareholders of an "S" corporation to allow the income, losses, and credits of the corporation to pass through to the shareholders, on a prorata basis the same way as in a partnership. For federal income tax purposes, this permits the shareholders to be taxed directly on the income earned by the corporation, making an "S" corporation tax neutral (in other words, the taxes are paid by individuals, not by the corporation) to its individual shareholders.

First, let's investigate why a person would choose to elect an "S" corporation rather than a typical or "C" corporation. An "S" corporation shareholder pays income taxes only once—at the individual income tax rates when the income is earned. A "C" corporation shareholder pays income taxes twice—the corporate tax rate when the income is earned and at the individual tax rate when the income is passed from the corporation to the individuals.

In order to evaluate the tax aspects of an "S" corporation, you must compare the tax rates for an individual with the tax rates of a "C" corporation since "S" corporation shareholders pay taxes at the individual tax return level only. To illustrate, let's assume you are a married physician who files a tax return jointly with your spouse. To begin, compare the tax rates of the married filing jointly tax schedule in Figure 2-1 with the corporate tax rates shown in Figure 2-2.

In comparing these rates for low levels of income, it initially appears as though a "C" corporation is better. For example, because you are taxed as an individual (using the tax rates in Figure 2-1) for the owner of an "S" corporation, the first $38,000 of income is taxed at a rate of 15 percent while a corporation has the 15 percent rate until its income surpasses $50,000. From $50,000 to $75,000 the corporate tax rate is 25 percent, while the married individuals' rate is 28 percent. To illustrate, a comparison of a corporation and an individual having taxable income of $75,000 follows:

| Married Individual | | Corporation | |
Taxable Income Range	Rate	Taxable Income Range	Rate
0 – $38,000	15%	0 – $50,000	15%
$38,000 – $75,000	28%	$50,000 – $75,000	25%
Total Tax – $16,060		Total Tax – $13,750	

With taxable income of $75,000, a married individual (using an "S" corporation) pays approximately 14 percent more income tax than a "C" corporation. This tax break at low profit levels was undoubtedly a scheme to aid the small business corporation when you note that the corporate tax rate leaps to 39 percent when taxable income exceeds $100,000, compared to 31 percent for the married individual.

However, at higher income levels, the "S" corporation which uses individual rates begins to show its superiority. Thus, at taxable income of $200,000, an individual pays $57,305 in taxes, while a corporation would pay $61,250. As a result, you can see that the beneficial tax structure depends upon your income level.

FIGURE 2-1
MARRIED FILING JOINTLY AND SURVIVING SPOUSES

Taxable Income Range	Pay	plus Percent	of the Amount Over
$ 0 – $ 38,000	$ 0	15%	$ 0
$ 38,000 – $ 91,850	$ 5,700.00	28%	$ 38,000
$ 91,850 – $140,000	$20,778.00	31%	$ 91,850
$140,000 – $250,000	$35,704.50	36%	$140,000
$250,000 –	$75,304.50	39.6%	$250,000

FIGURE 2-2
SELECT CORPORATE TAX RATES

Taxable Income Rate	But Not Over	Tax
0	$ 50,000	15%
$ 50,000	$ 75,000	25%
$ 75,000	$ 100,000	34%
$100,000	$ 335,000	39%
$335,000	$10,000,000	34%

However, the biggest problem with a "C" corporation is that when the profits from the corporation are distributed to the shareholders, the shareholders must pay individual taxes. Thus, "C" corporation shareholders are taxed twice: once with corporate taxes and once with individual income taxes. "S" corporation shareholders are taxed only once.

You must remember that the concept of limited liability remains unchanged because the "S" corporation election is an income tax concept and has nothing to do with the general legal concepts of the corporation. Many states have corporate income taxes and likewise, many states permit an "S" corporation election.

However, the "S" corporation has drawbacks, such as there cannot be more than 35 shareholders and none of the shareholders can be nonresident aliens. Shareholders must, with two limited exceptions, be natural persons and cannot be other business entities, such as a partnership or a corporation. However, certain qualified subchapter "S" trusts and estates may be a shareholder in an "S" corporation.

Professional Corporation (PC)

Next, we turn to the tax aspects of a PC. The Internal Revenue Code defines a "qualified personal service corporation" as any corporation that performs services in the fields of health, law, engineering, architecture, accounting, actuarial science, performing arts, and consulting. To qualify as a professional corporation, substantially all of the stock must be owned directly by the employees or retired employees who perform(ed) services for the corporation or their estates.

Unfortunately, the personal service corporation is not entitled to the graduated rates illustrated in the prior example. Rather, personal service corporations have a flat tax rate of 35 percent on all taxable income. You pay relatively high corporate tax rates on all income and then pay individual taxes if and when the profits are distributed to the shareholders. Therefore, from a tax point of view, you wouldn't select a corporation for the benefit of its graduated rates since they do not apply to a professional corporation.

Limited Liability Company (LLC)

The question of how the LLC will be taxed for federal income tax purposes is determined under federal law and not state law. An entity can be deemed to be a partnership for state law purposes but taxed as a corporation for federal tax purposes. The opposite is also true; an entity could be deemed a partnership for federal tax purposes and be taxed as a corporation for state law purposes. Therefore, in a particular state an LLC could be taxed as a partnership for federal income tax and as a corporation for state tax purposes. However, the states that have adopted LLC legislation have generally changed the state tax scheme so that the same type of tax is imposed at both the state and federal levels.

To determine if an entity will be taxed as a corporation or as a partnership, the Internal Revenue Service analyzes an LLC by certain criteria set forth in its regulations. These regulations set forth six basic characteristics necessary for the entity to be taxed as a corporation. They are:

- Associates
- Business purpose
- Continuity of life
- Centralized management
- Limited liability for corporate debts
- Free transferability of interest

Since both a partnership and a corporation will have associates and a business objective, the four remaining factors need to be considered.

The Internal Revenue Service has concluded that an LLC should be treated as a partnership for federal income tax purposes provided that it lacks at least two of the above four remaining corporate characteristics. Each state's statute and an LLC's Articles of Association will have to be examined to determine whether or not two of the four factors are lacking.

Now that we have examined the legal and tax aspects of each form of organization, we will conclude our discussion with a description of the advantages and disadvantages of each.

Advantages and Disadvantages of Each Form of Business Organization

Sole Proprietorship

To select this form of business organization for your medical practice is inexpensive. As a sole proprietor, you make all decisions and receive all profits, as well as incur all losses. Your earnings are taxed at your individual personal income tax rate.

As a sole proprietor, you receive no protection from personal liability and your personal assets are at risk. The growth of your practice is limited to your available resources.

Partnerships

A partnership allows a group of physicians to pool their financial resources and form a medical practice without a formal structure. Taxation of a partnership results in taxation to you as an individual, and therefore, has no impact on your individual tax result.

A general partnership does not enhance your protection from personal liability. Rather, it increases your potential personal liability because you may be obligated, as a partner, to a pay a verdict which arose without any fault on your part. Partnerships are terminable at will by any of the partners and the partnership is dissolved upon the death of a partner.

Limited Partnership

The limited partnership acts as a conduit for income tax purposes and provides limited liability to the extent of your investment in that business organization.

A limited partner is precluded from taking an active part in the management of the organization. To do so could subject the limited partner to unlimited liability equal to that of the general partner.

Corporation

Organizing your medical practice as a corporation provides limited liability and gives you the most protection for your personal assets. Unless the liability arises from one's own activity or one's agent, your only risk is to the extent of your investment in the stock of the corporation. The corporation is a separate legal entity, separate and distinct from you as an owner, and it may have perpetual life.

While a "C" corporation can gain the benefit of graduated corporate tax rates, a personal service corporation cannot and is taxed at a flat rate of 35 percent. An "S" corporation passes income and deductions directly to you the shareholders, and therefore, you are taxed at individual rates.

Thus, partnerships, limited partnerships, and "S" corporations are tax neutral from a federal income tax perspective, since they pass income and deductions directly to the individuals.

Limited Liability Company

If you organize as an LLC, your business assets will remain at risk to the extent of your investment in the LLC. The LLC taxes its members as individuals, and therefore, has no impact on your tax result. However, while the LLC is treated as a partnership for federal income tax purposes, it may not be recognized as such for state taxes and could be taxed as a corporation.

Physician's Checklist

As a summary of this chapter, ask yourself the following questions with respect to your medical practice. If you can answer "yes" to these questions, you have a good understanding of the legal and tax considerations affecting your medical practice.

_____ 1. Do you know which forms of organization protect your personal assets from the risks of the business?

_____ 2. Do you understand the different tax effects under the various forms of business organization?

_____ 3. Did you know that you can have personal liability, regardless of the form of business organization in which you operate your practice?

_____ 4. Are you aware that operating a business as a sole proprietor is the equivalent of operating the business as an individual?

_____ 5. Are you aware that operating as a general partnership gives you unlimited liability for your acts and the acts of your partners, while permitting you to be taxed as an individual?

_____ 6. Are you aware that a limited partnership limits your liability but allows you to be taxed as an individual?

_____ 7. Are you aware that the owners of a corporation have limited liability to the extent of their investment in the corporation?

_____ 8. Are you aware that an LLC, a relatively new form of business organization, now exists?

At the present time, most personal service groups are operating as professional corporations. Additional study will be required to determine if attorneys will recommend converting a personal service corporation into an LLC. We suggest that for the present, you continue with your professional corporation. Also, you should meet with your attorney and CPA prior to the close of each tax year for planning purposes and again after the close of the tax year for review purposes.

Now that you understand the role of your accountant and how and why your practice is organized from a legal and tax perspective, you are ready to begin the study and assessment of your financial results.

Questions and Answers

1. **What form of business organization provides the most asset protection?**

   The corporate form of organization provides the most asset protection.

2. **How is a proprietorship taxed?**

   The proprietorship is taxed directly to the individual.

3. **How is a partnership taxed?**

   The partnership itself is not taxed. The partnership files an informational return only and revenues and expenses flow directly from the partnership to the individual partner. The partner is then responsible for reporting that information on his or her personal tax return. This means that income from the medical practice is taxed at the individual rates of the partners.

4. **How is a corporation taxed?**

Corporations are taxed as a separate taxable entity using corporate tax rates.

5. **My medical practice is organized as an "S" corporation. How does this affect my income tax status?**

An "S" corporation passes income and deductions directly to you, the shareholders, and therefore you are taxed at individual rates.

6. **What is the newly emerging form of business organization known as an "LLC"?**

The new form of organization, an LLC, is a limited liability company. It combines the tax advantages of a partnership with the asset protection advantage of a corporation.

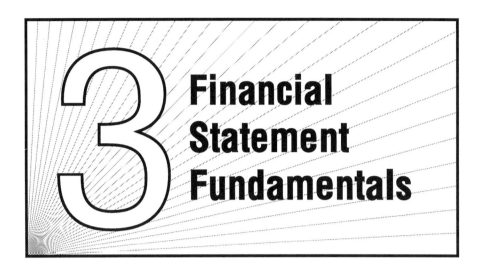

3 Financial Statement Fundamentals

Dr. R. M. Lave has a few spare minutes before he is scheduled to meet with his accountant to review his annual financial statements. Since he has now mastered the language of accounting and finance, and understands why his practice is organized as a professional corporation, he is feeling more comfortable with his financial affairs. As a result, he is determined to forge ahead! Thus, he begins a review of his financial statements prior to the meeting.

However, one issue leaves him puzzled. In reviewing his Statement of Revenues and Expenses, he notes that the practice showed a profit for the period. Yet, he distinctly remembered that the office manager told him earlier in the month that there wasn't enough cash to pay all of the suppliers whose bills were due at that time. He wonders how the practice could show a profit when, apparently, there wasn't enough cash to pay the bills. While considering that issue he turns to the Statement of Cash Flows and notes that the statement reports that more cash was paid out than the practice received during the period.

In looking for an answer to his question, Dr. Lave flips to the Statement of Assets, Liabilities and Equity and notices that there is, in fact, a reasonable balance in the cash account. However, he notices that the amount reported is actually lower than the cash balance from the prior period, but it appears to be adequate to meet the cash needs of the practice. Once again, he makes a note to ask the accountant to explain how they could have a profit and report a cash balance while available cash had been a problem.

The questions Dr. Lave raised are excellent ones and are the same questions faced by many businesses. Understanding your financial statement information and how it can help you answer these and other questions is a good start. Although you were briefly introduced to the financial statements in Chapter 1, they deserve an entire chapter for a full explanation of their uses and benefits to your medical practice. The questions Dr. Lave raised earlier can be answered with a thorough explanation of your financial results.

This chapter is going to answer the question of profit or income, versus cash flows, and other frequently asked questions on financial statements. Specifically, this chapter will address:

- What is the purpose of financial statements?
- What are the financial statements and what information do they provide?
- How and when are financial statements prepared?
- Why is there a difference between profit and cash flow?
- What should you do with your financial statements when you receive them?
- What role do the financial statements play in managing your practice?

In order to follow the discussion closely, sample financial statements of a medical practice have been provided in Figures 3-1 through 3-4. Reference to these illustrations throughout the discussion will be helpful. We also highly recommend that you use the most recent copy of your own financial statements, compare them to the illustration, and refer to them frequently during the following discussion.

The Purpose of Financial Statements

Financial statements actually have many purposes. However, the most significant one is that they **summarize** the events that took place in your medical practice. Because they are the end product of the accounting cycle (see Chapter 1), they are the sum total of each and every financial transaction that occurred. Thus, any and all events that affected revenue, expense, asset, liability or equity accounts, are represented in the financial statements.

Another purpose of financial statements is that they **group** like transactions together. This allows you to see the net impact of all related financial transactions during a specified period. Because they group similar transactions into a single figure, you obtain the needed financial information without the volumes of detail that underlie each balance. This normally suffices unless there is a specific need for such detailed information in managing your medical practice.

Further, the financial statements represent a **standard presentation** of your financial transactions. While this may not seem important, it actually helps you assess the results of your practice because it is in the same prescribed form each and every period. Thus, once you master the presentation mechanics, you can simply focus on what is important in the financial statements (i.e., the numerical results).

In addition, a quick glance at the form of presentation allows you to quickly identify anything that is different in a given period. A further benefit of the standard prescribed format is its comparability among medical practices. If you are considering a partnership with other physicians and obtain their financial statements, you will see the same information, in the same order, as your statements.

Focused Feedback on your medical practice is another important purpose provided by financial statements. As you get caught up in your day-to-day activities, it is easy to overlook the business side of your practice. Receiving financial statements periodically gives you the prompting needed to focus on the financial side of your business at regular intervals. This focused feedback, coupled with the standard presentation described earlier, easily gives you the information you need.

In summary, prudent use of your financial statements will highlight critical information, allowing you to plan for changing conditions, or events that need further attention. One note of caution is necessary, however. Remember that a financial statement represents a summary of past information; using it as a prescription for the future is not always wise.

Financial Statements

There are four standard financial statements, although many physicians receive only the first three with their accountant's report. The financial statements are: (1) a Statement of Assets, Liabilities and Equity, (2) the Statement of Revenues and Expenses, (3) the Statement of Shareholders' Equity, and (4) the Statement of Cash Flows. The most commonly omitted financial statement is the Statement of Cash Flows. After reading the material in this chapter and Chapter 5, you may want to ask your accountant to include this financial statement with the others in his or her report.

The financial statements appear together as a package and it is important to view them as one because of the interrelationships that exist. The interrelationships among the first three statements were identified and discussed in Chapter 1, and illustrated in Figure 1-2. Because of these interrelationships, examining a single financial statement is of limited value.

The Statement of Assets, Liabilities and Equity

The Statement of Assets, Liabilities and Equity, illustrated in Figure 3-1, shows the financial resources, debts, and ownership interest in the practice at a particular point in time.

Before you review the formal statement of your medical practice, the main idea and purpose of the Statement of Assets, Liabilities and Equity can be illustrated with the simple example of purchasing your personal residence with a mortgage. The asset you acquire (a house) was obtained by borrowing from the bank (a mortgage) and any down payment you made (your equity). Thus, if this is your only financial transaction, your personal Statement of Assets, Liabilities and Equity would look like the following:

ASSETS	=	LIABILITIES	+	OWNER'S EQUITY
Personal Residence		Mortgage		Personal Funds Contributed

FIGURE 3-1
R. M. LAVE, PROFESSIONAL CORPORATION
STATEMENT OF ASSETS, LIABILITIES AND EQUITY
MODIFIED CASH BASIS
DECEMBER 31, 1994

	1994	1993

ASSETS
    CURRENT ASSETS
        Cash
        Marketable Securities
        Notes Receivable
        Prepaid Insurance
        Prepaid Taxes
        Deposits
        Supplies Inventory
    TOTAL CURRENT ASSETS
    PROPERTY AND EQUIPMENT
        Land
        Building
        Equipment
        Furniture and Fixtures
        Leasehold Improvements
        Vehicles
            Less: Accumulated Depreciation
    TOTAL PROPERTY AND EQUIPMENT
    OTHER ASSETS
        Restrictive Covenants
        Goodwill
    TOTAL OTHER ASSETS
TOTAL ASSETS

LIABILITIES AND SHAREHOLDERS' EQUITY
    CURRENT LIABILITIES
        Notes Payable
        Payroll Taxes Withheld
        Income Taxes Payable
        Mortgage Payables—Current Portion
        Accrued Pension
        Line of Credit
    TOTAL CURRENT LIABILITIES
    LONG-TERM LIABILITIES
        Notes Payable (net of current portion)
        Mortgage Payable (net of current portion)
    TOTAL LONG-TERM LIABILITIES
    TOTAL LIABILITIES
    SHAREHOLDERS' EQUITY
        Common Stock
          $10 par value, 5,000 shares
          authorized, 2,000 issued
        Additional Paid-in Capital
        Retained Earnings
          Less: Treasury Stock 500
            shares at cost
    TOTAL SHAREHOLDERS' EQUITY
TOTAL LIABILITIES AND SHAREHOLDERS' EQUITY

With this personal statement, you can see how the acquisition of the asset was financed with a combination of bank borrowing and your down payment. Thus, your equity interest at this point is equal to the amount of personal funds you invested.

The Statement of Assets, Liabilities and Equity for your practice works the same way and shows the same type of information; it is just on a larger scale.

The other common name for this financial statement is the *balance sheet*, which is the title used by other types of business operations. Perhaps it would be helpful to think of your Statement of Assets, Liabilities, and Equity simply as a balance sheet, keeping in mind that the balance sheet is appropriately named and therefore must "balance." This simply means that your firm's assets or resources must balance with the combination of the debts of your practice and the ownership interests. That is why the balance sheet number, "total assets," will always equal the sum of the numbers of the total liabilities and total shareholders or partners' equity.

A Statement of Assets, Liabilities and Equity for a medical practice is illustrated in Figure 3-1. In trying to understand it, just remember that it is nothing more than the sum of many transactions similar to purchasing your home.

The Statement of Assets, Liabilities and Equity is normally the first financial statement presented in your accountant's report. This statement reports your financial information only at **one particular point** in time. However, you also need to receive information that reports on the **activities** of the practice **over a period of time**. This reporting is accomplished with the remaining three financial statements. Our discussion will begin with the Statement of Revenues and Expenses.

The Statement of Revenues and Expenses and Shareholders' Equity

The Statement of Revenue and Expenses, illustrated in Figure 3-2, is appropriately titled since it reports the total revenues your practice has generated over a specific period of time. It also reports the amount of expenses in the same time period. The resulting difference between the two is called net income. *Net* simply means after all expenses have been accounted for; *income* means with the presumption that the revenues will, in fact, exceed expenses. If this is not actually the case, a net loss is reported.

Once again, the purpose of this statement can be illustrated with an example using a month of your personal income and expenses. The amount of *revenue* would be equal to the value of your take-home paycheck while your *operating expenses* are nothing more than your cash outlay for expenses during the month.

REVENUE	=	TAKE-HOME PAYCHECK
LESS: OPERATING EXPENSES	=	UTILITIES
		PROPERTY TAXES
		INTEREST ON MORTGAGE
		FOOD
		CLOTHES
		MISCELLANEOUS
NET INCOME		EXCESS OF PAYCHECK OVER EXPENSES

The Statement of Revenues and Expenses for your practice works the same way and shows the same information; it is just on a larger scale. The Statement of Revenues and Expenses, often called the Income Statement by other types of businesses, is illustrated in Figure 3-2.

FIGURE 3-2
R. M. LAVE, PROFESSIONAL CORPORATION
STATEMENT OF REVENUES AND EXPENSES
MODIFIED CASH BASIS
FOR THE YEARS ENDED DECEMBER 31, 1994 AND 1993

	1994	1993
REVENUES		
Fees		
Less: Refunds		
NET PATIENT REVENUES		
OPERATING EXPENSES		
Wages and Salaries—Physicians		
Wages and Salaries—Staff		
Medical Supplies		
Rent		
Employee Benefits		
Payroll Taxes		
Office Supplies		
Utilities		
Auto Expenses		
Rent		
Professional Seminars		
TOTAL OPERATING EXPENSES		
ADMINISTRATIVE EXPENSES		
Insurance		
Professional Fees		
Maintenance and Repairs		
Depreciation		
Interest Expense		
Dues and Subscriptions		
TOTAL ADMINISTRATIVE EXPENSES		
INCOME FROM OPERATIONS		
OTHER REVENUES/EXPENSE		
Interest Revenue		
Rental Revenue		
INCOME BEFORE TAXES		
Income Tax Expense		
NET INCOME		

The amount of profit shown as net income is transferred from the Statement of Revenues and Expenses to the Statement of Shareholders' (or Partners') Equity. You can think of this as the excess of your paycheck over expenses being subsequently deposited in your personal savings account. That is, the excess represents an addition to your savings balance.

Thus, if you want to know how much you could save, you would look at your Statement of Revenues and Expenses. If you want to see how and when the deposit would increase your personal account, you would look at the Statement of Changes in Equity; and if you wanted to know the balance in your savings account after the deposit, you would examine the Statement of Assets, Liabilities and Equity. These relationships are illustrated below.

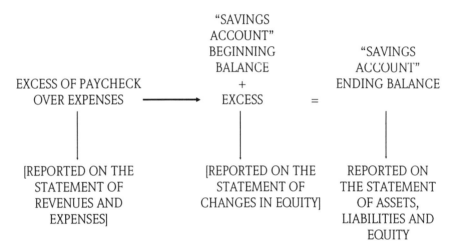

Thus, the connecting link between the Statement of Revenues and Expenses, with the ultimate placement of net income into retained earnings or a partner's capital account, is shown on the Statement of Changes in Shareholders' Equity, illustrated in Figure 3-3.

Although the entire statement appears below, only the retained earnings balance is affected by the reporting of net income. The stock and additional paid-in capital accounts are only affected when a buy-in or buy-out occurs. However, they are included in this presentation so that you can see a complete financial statement.

In a partnership or proprietorship, this statement is actually much simpler. The retained earnings account is replaced by the owner's individual capital account and the other accounts are nonexistent. Thus, net income or net losses increase/decrease the owner's capital account directly.

The Statement of Cash Flows

The fourth statement, the Statement of Cash Flows, is an important statement for physicians because cash flow concerns are often critical in the management of a medical

FIGURE 3-3
R. M. LAVE, PROFESSIONAL CORPORATION
STATEMENTS OF SHAREHOLDERS' EQUITY
MODIFIED CASH BASIS
FOR THE YEARS ENDED DECEMBER 31, 1994 AND 1993

	Retained Earnings	Common Stock Shares	Common Stock Amount	Additional Paid-in Capital
Balance, January 1, 1993				
Net loss	–			
Balance, December 31, 1993				
Net income, 1994	–			
Balance, December 31, 1994				

practice. This statement, illustrated in Figure 3-4, takes all cash inflows for the firm, and all cash outflows for the firm, and categorizes them into one of three activities:

- Operating Activities from the primary business purpose
- Investing Activities; those where you invest in the assets used by the medical practice, such as the purchase of equipment
- Financing Activities; which describe how you financed the medical practice (i.e., either through borrowed money or through additional investment by the physicians)

To help you understand this statement, consider the preparation of a Statement of Cash Flows on a personal level. Your cash inflow (i.e., paycheck) would be listed as an operating activity. You must then analyze your cash payments for the month and classify each check according to the nature of the transaction. A personal operating activity would be for such items as food and utilities; *investing activities* reflect your investment in personal long-lived assets (i.e., the purchase of a house, car, or furniture); while the *financing activities* would illustrate how you paid for those items (i.e., a bank loan for the car or a mortgage on the house).

A Statement of Cash Flows for a medical practice is illustrated in Figure 3-4.

This statement also connects to the other financial statements since it uses net income from the Statement of Revenues and Expenses as its starting point and concludes with the same cash balance that is reported on the Statement of Assets, Liabilities and Equity. To see how the Statement of Cash Flows interrelates with the other financial statements, Figure 1-2 has been restated in Figure 3-5 to illustrate the connection with the fourth financial statement.

FIGURE 3-4
STATEMENT OF CASH FLOWS
MODIFIED CASH BASIS
FOR THE YEARS ENDED DECEMBER 31, 1994 AND 1993

CASH FLOWS FROM OPERATING ACTIVITIES
    Net Income
    Adjustments to Reconcile Net Income to Net
      Cash Provided by Operating Activities:
        Depreciation
        Amortization
        (Increase) Decrease in Prepaid Income Taxes
        Increase (Decrease) in Payroll Taxes Withheld
        Increase in Income Taxes Payable

          Net Cash Provided by Operating Activities

CASH FLOWS FROM INVESTING ACTIVITIES:
    Purchase of Office Furniture and Equipment

          Net Cash Flows (Used) by Investing Activities

CASH FLOWS FROM FINANCING ACTIVITIES:
    Repayment of Notes Payable
    Payments on Mortgage Payable
          Net Cash Flows (Used) by Financing Activities

          Net (Decrease) in Cash

CASH—BEGINNING OF YEAR

CASH—END OF YEAR

SUPPLEMENTAL DISCLOSURES:

    Total Cash Paid for:
        Income Taxes
        Interest

FIGURE 3-5
FINANCIAL STATEMENT INTERRELATIONSHIPS

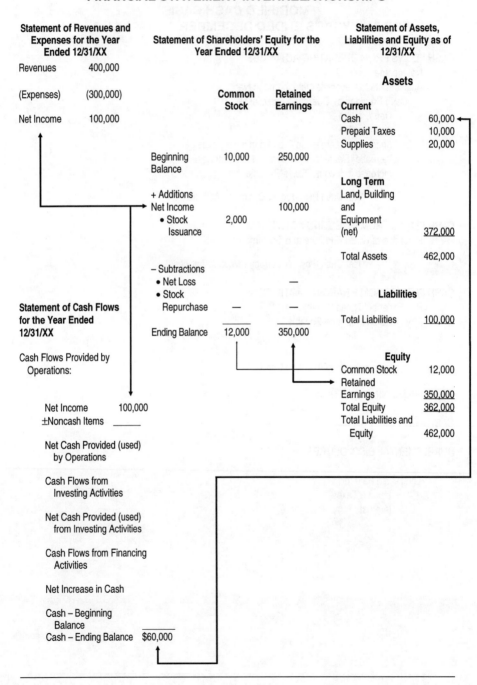

How and When Are Financial Statements Prepared?

Depending on the financial reporting needs of your practice, financial statements can be prepared as frequently as monthly, quarterly (at the end of any three-month period), or annually. Most medical practices receive quarterly reports from their accountant, followed by annual reports at year end. For timely financial management of your medical practice, monthly financial reporting is highly recommended. Although your accountant may not prepare monthly statements, the required information is readily available in your accounting system.

Financial statement data are obtained from the transactions processed in the accounting cycle and statements cannot be prepared unless all accounting information for the period has been processed. The required information includes the accounting cycle elements identified in Chapter 1. Thus, the journal entries that record daily activity, the journal entries that record the needed periodic adjustments, such as for medical supplies used from inventory, as well as the closing journal entries which finalize the financial reporting for the period, must be considered. If you are still unclear as to how this process works, please refer back to the section entitled Accounting Records in Chapter 1.

The financial statements can be prepared by your practice's accountant, if you employ one, or by the office manager, if they have the necessary background to do so. This requires, however, that the individual also perform the adjusting and closing process described in Chapter 1. Many small to mid-size practices do not have an individual who can perform this function, so they rely on their outside accountant to perform these tasks.

Whether you choose to have your financial statements prepared on a monthly basis, rather than a quarterly or annual basis, is a decision that you must make. However, for sound financial management, it is better to focus on your financial results on a timely basis. Therefore, you should consider using either an employee or an outside accountant to produce the required accounting information. If you do not employ an accountant or you are concerned with the fees paid for accounting services, a Statement of Revenues and Expenses for the period, in lieu of the entire financial statement package, could be prepared. This has some obvious limitations, however, and should only be considered as a last resort.

It is also important to note that preparation of the current financial statements is of little help for management purposes unless the prior period's financial information is also presented. For example, to learn that fees for the current month were $80,000 doesn't necessarily give you much information on the practice. However, if you also know that your fees for the same time period last year were $52,000, or in contrast, $96,000, you receive very different feedback. Thus, comparative information is a must when preparing and reviewing financial information.

Basis of Preparation

As we discussed in Chapter 1, your accountant's report refers to the financial statements *basis* of preparation. This reference tells you the underlying method of financial recording and dictates when you record financial transactions in the accounting records. Most accountant's reports for medical practices refer to financial statements prepared on a cash basis, a modified cash basis, or an income tax basis. Regardless of what it is called, these three methods consider the same financial statement elements.

In order to understand what it means, however, it is helpful to understand the basis of preparation that is not often used in medical practice accounting systems, namely the accrual basis. This is useful because the basis most commonly referred to in your accountant's report (i.e., cash, modified cash, or income tax basis) only uses cash basis reporting as a starting point. However, for certain financial statement elements, such as depreciation of equipment, the accrual basis system of recording is used. In addition, the question of cash flow versus net income, can only be answered if one thoroughly understands the differences between cash basis and accrual basis accounting.

Before we begin the specific discussion of cash versus accrual accounting, it is important to recognize two important facts. First, whatever the basis of preparation used in your medical practice, it must be consistently applied from one period to the next. Not only is this a requirement for sound financial reporting, it is also required by the Internal Revenue Service (IRS) for income tax reporting.

Second, you must understand that the basis of preparation for the medical practice can be different from that of your personal income tax return. Individuals are required by the IRS to prepare their personal tax returns on a cash basis, while the financial information of a medical practice can use any of the bases referred to above.

Cash Basis Accounting

A "pure" cash basis of accounting is actually the simplest in terms of preparation because the only time a transaction is recorded is when cash is received or paid. Thus, it is clear cut. If cash wasn't received or paid, no accounting entry is recorded in the accounting system.

This is not to say that your practice does not maintain a record of who owes you money for services. Rather, this information is not reported as revenue or income in the accounting system (via a journal entry, as shown in Chapter 1), until you actually receive the cash.

In fact, all medical practices maintain some form of an accounts receivable system for the amounts owed to the practice. However, accounts receivable will not feed into the reporting system that generates the financial statements if you are on a cash basis of accounting. (This is in contrast to accounts receivable records for an accrual based system, which are an integral part of the financial accounting and reporting system.)

Likewise, there is no recording of expenses until cash or a check is used to make payment. Although you may have received your utility bill in mid-January for December's usage, it is not a recorded expense until you pay the bill, even if it is in February.

It is interesting to note that the "pure" cash basis is not frequently used, even if it is referred to in your accountant's report. Rather, it is the modified cash basis that is used. Modified cash basis and income tax basis are essentially the same method of preparation since these methods use the basics of the cash method described above and combine it with the accrual method of accounting for certain financial statement elements. Therefore, we will examine the accrual basis of accounting before we discuss the modified cash or income tax basis.

Accrual Basis Accounting

Accrual accounting uses a different focus from cash basis accounting. Income is recorded whenever services are *earned* and expenses are recorded whenever they are *incurred.* Services are considered earned whenever you perform the necessary procedures for the patient and you can determine the amount due. In contrast, expenses are recorded whenever goods or services have been provided to your practice, even if you don't pay the bill until 60 days later.

If a medical practice is under an accrual rather than a cash basis system, information would be recorded differently (i.e., the revenues for services earned would be recorded the same day that you saw the patient). Likewise, the utility bill mentioned earlier would be recorded as a December expense even though it will be paid in a subsequent month.

Another example of accrual accounting concerns items purchased by the medical practice whose benefits carry over to more than one accounting period. For example, the purchase of equipment by the practice usually results in the creation of an equipment account which is an asset shown on the Statement of Assets, Liabilities and Equity. However, that equipment is used in providing the services which allow you to earn income. Thus, if you want to record the real cost of doing business in a certain time period, the expense of using the equipment must also be recognized. This is actually accomplished by transferring a portion of the cost of the equipment to an expense account for each period that the equipment is used.

Likewise, if your practice purchases medical supplies in bulk, they may not be used immediately, and may actually be consumed over a long period of time. Even though you paid for the supplies at one time, the cost of the supplies must be allocated to the time when they are used. Thus, accrual accounting records expenses, regardless of when they are paid, in the time period in which they are used.

You may wonder why the accrual system is used, given the simplicity of the cash system where the receipt or payment of cash determines when to record financial information. Although the cash basis system is by far the simplest, it is also subject to manipulation (e.g., by delaying the receipt or payment of cash, you can easily alter the reporting results of your business). To illustrate the impact cash versus accrual accounting can have, consider the simplified example in Figure 3-6.

Modified Cash or Income Tax Basis of Accounting

By now, you should understand the differences between cash and accrual accounting, and it should be easier to see how modified cash or income tax basis statements are prepared. A modified cash method takes the basic guidelines of cash basis (i.e., items are recorded whenever cash is received or paid) but adds the accrual basis guidelines for certain financial statement elements. These elements are: depreciation of building,

FIGURE 3-6
CASH VERSUS ACCRUAL BASIS OF ACCOUNTING

FACTS:

(1)	Dollar Value of Services Provided This Period	$ 80,000
(2)	Cash Received from Patients and Insurance Companies	$100,000
(3)	Cash Paid for Purchase of Medical Supplies	$ 4,000
(4)	Amount of Medical Supplies Used This Period	$ 1,000
(5)	Depreciation of Equipment	$ 6,000
(6)	Utility Bills Paid	$ 500
(7)	Utility—Actual Usage This Period	$ 600

Cash Basis Accounting (i.e., cash-in, cash-out)

Revenue	$100,000
Expenses:	
Medical Supplies	$ 4,000
Utilities	500
Net Income	$ 95,500

Accrual Basis Accounting (i.e., revenues when "earned," expenses when "incurred"):

Revenue	$ 80,000
Expenses:	
Medical Supplies	$ 1,000
Utilities	600
Depreciation	$ 6,000
Net Income	$ 72,400

equipment, and vehicles; the purchase of insurance policies whose coverage exceeds one year; rent of facilities paid in advance; and the use of medical or office supply inventories.

Using the facts from the illustration in Figure 3-6, a modified cash basis would produce the results shown in Figure 3-7.

You might wonder what all of this means to you, the medical practitioner, trying to understand your financial statements. Simply, that the Statement of Revenues and Expenses shows information that is recorded because it affects your cash account, and it shows expenses that did not affect the current period cash account. That is why there is a difference between cash flow and net income!

Net income considers expenses, such as depreciation, that actually affect cash flows in a different period. If you purchased equipment five years ago, the purchasing decision impacted cash flow at that time, but did not reduce net income in the year of purchase.

FIGURE 3-7
MODIFIED CASH BASIS ACCOUNTING

Modified Cash Basis:

Revenue	$100,000
Expenses:	
Medical Supplies	1,000
Utilities	500
Depreciation	6,000
Net Income	$ 92,500

Rather, the cost of the equipment is subsequently prorated over time and recorded as a current period expense corresponding with its usage. It is at this time that you will see a decrease in net income. However, depreciation expense does not affect cash flow in the year that the equipment is used.

Now that you know the basic facts of financial statement preparation, it is time to consider the question of what you should do when you receive the information.

What Should I Do with My Financial Statement Information?

Before we discuss what you should do with your financial statement information, it is better to suggest what you shouldn't do with it. First, you shouldn't just glance at the statements and put them in a file cabinet. This defeats the purpose of having them prepared. Second, you should not focus solely on one or two items. Financial statements need to be examined together as a total package. Focusing on an isolated item, such as net income, or on any one statement, will not only not provide you with the financial information you need to manage your practice, it can actually mislead you. Third, you should not assume that the accountant knows all of the information and therefore you don't need to take an active role in the process. It is your medical practice, your financial information, to be used by you, in making financial decisions.

One of the first things you should do with the financial statements is make sure that you understand what they are telling you, and just as importantly, what they don't. For example, because medical practices are on a cash or modified cash basis reporting (see the previous section), a significant financial element does not appear on your financial statements, specifically Accounts Receivable (i.e., the amount owed to you from patients and their insurance companies). Therefore, it is important to remember that this vital operating information must be incorporated into any discussion of the financial health of your practice.

The second thing you must do with the financial statements is get your partners involved! This is often difficult because of the daily demands of the practice, or because many practices designate one partner as the business manager of the practice. However, it is important that everyone involved in the practice understand the financial results. Sit down together and review them, both before and after the accountant meets with you. Not only will this help facilitate everyone's understanding in the short term, it will also help when it is time to make management decisions. Only when everyone has current knowledge and a similar information base from which to analyze the financial affairs of the practice, will efficient and effective decision making result.

You may think the above ideas are great in theory, but other than reading the financials and seeing a lot of numbers, what is there to talk about? Before you sit down to discuss the information with your associates, it is important to "get a handle on" the financial information provided in the standard format of the statements. There are several ways that you can do this, each involving translations of the financial statement information.

The next few pages will detail two concepts: (1) the use of percentage figures rather than dollar figures and (2) the use of trend analysis and other criteria for comparison.

Common-Size It!

Do you ever think about your personal financial situation and wonder where your money goes every month? Or did you ever wonder why a bank asks for a specific listing of your personal assets and debt obligations when you apply for a mortgage?

The answers to both of these questions lie in determining one specific financial element to your total financial picture. To illustrate, do you know how much of your monthly income is consumed by a particular expense (e.g., what percentage of your take-home pay is spent for food—1 percent, 5 percent, or more)? Or, how much of your resources are tied up in physical assets (cars, houses) as opposed to liquid assets (cash, certificates of deposit, etc.) available to pay off debts?

To answer these questions, you can restate your personal information on a relative basis. That is, divide each of your monthly operating expenses by the amount of your take-home pay and you will easily see what percent of your pay is consumed by each individual expense. Assume a take-home pay of $9,000 per month and utilities of $500, food and entertainment of $2,000, property taxes of $300, and insurances of $250. Of course, your mortgage is a significant outlay, but it is part expense (i.e., interest) and part principal (i.e., repayment of the debt). Therefore, we are excluding this in our expense analysis for simplification. Relating each of these expenses to the total shows that utilities are 5.5 percent ($500/9,000), food and entertainment are 22.2 percent ($2,000/9,000), property taxes 3.3 percent ($300/9,000), and insurances 2.78 percent ($250/9,999).

You can perform a similar analysis on your assets and debt as well. If the total assets you own are $800,000 and your house is valued at $400,000, it means that 50 percent of your available resources are tied up with the house. If you also consider that the mortgage debt is $300,000, medical school loans are $70,000, and credit card debt is

$20,000, it means that 48.75 percent ($390,000/800,000) of your assets are financed with debt as opposed to your equity interest, and 95 percent of your debt is long-term (i.e., due after one year) ($370,000/390,000).

A similar analysis is typically performed for business operations. To common-size your financial statements, often called vertical analysis, you simply translate the raw numerical information into results that show each financial statement on a relative basis. This translation shows how any individual number relates to the total and to each other within the statement. This is done in the same way we illustrated with your personal financial information (i.e., restating each element of a financial statement to a percentage of a particular number, for example, salaries as a percentage of patient fees).

Common-Sizing the Statement of Revenue and Expense

In fact, your accountant's report often shows some common-size data. Looking at your financial statements, you will often see a percentage next to the dollar value shown for each expense element on the Statement of Revenues and Expenses. This information assumes that fees, like your take-home paycheck in our earlier example, are 100 percent and it tells you what percentage of fees was consumed by each individual expense. Any significant change in this relative information warrants your further attention. To illustrate, if salaries as a percentage of patient fees increased from 32 percent to 40 percent in a given period, it would be smart to determine whether this change was caused by declining fees, increased salaries, the hiring of additional personnel, or more importantly, a combination of various factors.

Although the Statement of Revenues and Expenses is typically common-sized relative to the total fees, it is also helpful to examine the expense components, not as a basis of fees, but on a basis of total expenses. Knowing the expenses that constitute the most significant costs of your practice can help you when you are trying to make operating decisions. For example, if you determine that you must reduce your monthly operating costs, a logical place to begin is with the most significant cost. Therefore, if you know employee wages and salaries (excluding physicians) are 25 percent of your total operating budget, cutting costs in this area will have a greater impact than cutting costs in other areas.

Understanding the Nature of Costs

Medical practices must be managed as a business enterprise. However, this is difficult because of a lack of understanding about the interrelationships among cost components in a medical practice. By interrelationships, we mean how changes in one financial element cause corresponding changes in other related elements. For example, the decision to increase office hours will most notably cause an increase in wage and salary expense. However, it will also cause payroll taxes, supplies, and utilities to increase. In contrast, it will not cause an increase in expenses such as malpractice insurance or depreciation. This is due to the nature of the costs involved.

Therefore, you also need a fundamental understanding of the *nature* of your cost elements. By nature, we mean the type of costs and how they change when other factors, such as increased office hours, change. It is difficult to determine the appropriate course of action in the decision-making process, without understanding cost structure and the relationships among costs and revenues.

It is a mistake to regard operating expenses in the same way. In reality, there are three types of expenses and each one reacts differently to operating changes in the practice. These three types of expenses are: *fixed*, which do not vary with changes in the level of operations; *variable*, which change directly with changes in the level of operations; and *semivariable costs*, which contain some fixed and some variable components.

An example of a fixed cost is malpractice insurance. Its rate does not increase with a higher patient load. In contrast, a variable cost can be illustrated with medical supplies (i.e., the more patients you see, the more supplies are consumed and the higher your expenses).

Nursing staff can be classified as semivariable. Although you can probably see several extra patients with the existing staffing level, any major increase in new patient volume or hours would most likely require the addition of a staff person. Thus, you can think of this cost as a "step" cost (i.e., at each level of cost, there is a range of patients that can be seen). This occurs until you hit a maximum load, at which time staff hours must be added and therefore additional costs incurred in order to continue increasing the patient contact volume or hours.

Thus, when considering operating changes in the practice, it is beneficial to know how expenses will change as a result. Understanding the nature of the expense item and recognizing that a given cost element may represent a substantial portion of your total operating expenses, is a good start. It is also important, however, to examine these changes over time. Therefore, you must also perform a trend analysis (see the next section in this chapter) for further information.

Common-Sizing the Statement of Assets, Liabilities and Equity

Additional information is also readily available if you prepare a common-size Statement of Assets, Liabilities and Equity, at least on an occasional basis. This is the same process used in our personal assets and liabilities described earlier. You might ask, why? Consider the example for business assets noted in Figure 3-8; this readily highlights certain information when shown in common-size terms.

What the common-size information in Figure 3-8 easily and clearly demonstrates is that the asset base for each of these practices is quite different. Note that in dollar terms, the property and equipment of Firms B and C are not that different. However, the percentage of business assets consumed by this type of assets is substantially different.

In addition, you can see that while Firm B has a relative balance between liquid (i.e., current assets) and long-term assets, Firm A has a significant amount of assets in a highly liquid state. In contrast, Firm C has almost 90 percent of their assets invested in property and equipment.

Although there may be various reasons why these practices have the specific asset components they do, Figure 3-8 clearly highlights the type of asset base each firm has and the potential problems that may exist as a result. For example, there may be limits

FIGURE 3-8
COMMON-SIZE ASSET INFORMATION

	Firm A		Firm B		Firm C	
	$	%	$	%	$	%
Current Assets	102,200	73	84,800	53	13,000	13
Property and Equipment (net)	37,800	27	75,200	47	87,000	87
TOTAL ASSETS	140,000	100	160,000	100	100,000	100

to the financial flexibility of Firm C since 90 percent of their asset base is in fixed assets. These assets may not be readily marketable and may, in fact, be difficult to convert into cash in the event of needed cash flow.

For businesses other than medical practices, this type of information is typically compared to standard industry ratios. At present, there is no such information readily available to medical practices. However, there is still a benefit to preparing a common-size analysis for your own firm so that this type of information is not overlooked. It will also be a useful analysis in cases where a merger of two practices is pending.

One final note regarding common-size financial statements. Just as a single financial statement is of limited value, common-size information must also be prepared and analyzed for a minimum of two accounting periods.

Trend Analysis

Trend analysis, often called horizontal analysis, examines your financial statement elements over a period of time. This analysis is performed for each account by calculating the dollar difference in a two-year period and restating the difference in percentage terms, using the first year as the base. Thus, if revenues increase from $80,000 to $90,000 from year one to year two, the calculation would be $10,000/80,000 or a 12½ percent increase.

Trend analysis is normally prepared for a minimum of a three- to five-year period. Only with this expanded time line will the information be of benefit. However, actual preparation of the information is only the first step. Analysis and interpretation is the second step and planning for needed changes is the third.

Determining the cause of the change is essential. In addition, you must examine the related accounts to see if the corresponding changes in those accounts make sense. For example, assume that fees earned increased 12½ percent from year one to year two. Identifying the reason for the increase is important and one must consider whether or not the increase was due to one specific change or a combination of events. Logical reasons for the increases might be: increases in fee structure, offering additional office hours, increases in volume of existing patients, or acquisition of new patients during the year.

Depending on the answer to the question of why revenues increased, you must then examine the related costs. For example, if the increase in revenues was caused by adding new office hours in the evening to better serve your patients, increases in related expenses for such items as utilities, wage and salary expense, and office or medical supplies would be expected. If revenues increased $12\frac{1}{2}$ percent from year one to year two, and the expenses in these categories only increased 4 percent, it is easy to see that the incremental revenues exceed the incremental costs on a relative basis. Therefore, the additional hours represent a sound operating decision. More information on trend analysis is presented in Chapter 5, Operating Information.

It is easy to recognize that not all decisions in a medical practice can be made on the basis of a simple numerical analysis. However, this information must be considered when making operating decisions. Also remember that trend analysis should be prepared for a minimum of three to five years. This allows you to focus on the long-term changes that affect your practice. This information, coupled with the common-size data and the current financial statement information, gives you, the physician, the necessary information needed to manage your medical practice.

The Role of Financial Statements in Managing a Medical Practice

Although the discussion in this chapter has focused on the mechanics of financial statements, how they are prepared, their basis of preparation, and what you should do when you receive the information, it is beneficial to revisit the role financial statements play in managing your medical practice.

First and foremost is the feedback that the financial statements give. Their results show you the "big picture" of all individual operating transactions. We recognize that it is virtually impossible for a physician to assess and evaluate the results of a medical practice on a daily basis. It is not necessary that the physician manage every minute detail of the medical practice. What is important, however, is that the physician understand the impact of the daily activities and individual transactions. It is in this venue that the financial statements serve a vital role. Presenting the big picture reduces the critical operating information needed for sound decision making to a manageable level of detail.

The second role that financial statements serve in a medical practice is acting as a focal point. By receiving the financial statements on a periodic basis, you should naturally be compelled to focus on the financial results of the practice. This role is actually two sided in that it allows you to have in-depth discussions with your partners in the practice, as well as have knowledgeable discussions with accountants, bankers, or others with a vested interest in your business.

The third role financial statements serve in managing a medical practice is the assessment role. Receiving and subsequently analyzing your financial statements gives you all the necessary information to assess the results of your operation. It also helps you to determine where changes need to be made and what the changes should be. Again, a word of caution in this area: the assessment mechanism is important but it does focus on past information. Its restrictive usefulness in projecting future results must always be recognized.

In summary, the role financial statements play in managing a medical practice is one of information. Without the data and subsequent analysis of the results, physicians would be making decisions virtually blind. Thus, never underestimate the value of financial statement information in managing your medical practice.

Physician's Checklist

As a summary of this chapter, ask yourself the following questions with respect to your medical practice. If you can answer "yes" to these questions, you have a good understanding of financial statement fundamentals.

_____ 1. Do you know which financial statements you receive from your accountant?

_____ 2. Do you understand the purpose of each of these statements?

_____ 3. Do you understand the interrelationships between your financial statements?

_____ 4. Do you know when and how often your financial statements are prepared?

_____ 5. Are your statements prepared frequently enough to serve your needs?

_____ 6. Do you know the basis on which your statements are prepared and do you understand the underlying assumptions of that method?

_____ 7. Do you restate your financial statements on a common-size basis?

_____ 8. Do you perform trend analysis on your financial statement data?

_____ 9. Do you use your financial statements as an assessment tool and promptly evaluate the results of your medical practice?

Understanding the financial statement fundamentals discussed in this chapter gives you the necessary information to consider other, more in-depth, aspects of each of the four financial statements. Chapter 4 begins this process with a detailed discussion of the Statement of Assets, Liabilities and Equity.

Questions and Answers

1. **How are financial statements interrelated?**

   The financial statement package begins with net income reported on the Statement of Revenues and Expenses. From there, net income is transferred to the Statement of Changes in Shareholders' Equity (or the Statement of

Partner's or Owner's Capital, in other than a corporate form of organization). Once the net income amount is transferred to the Statement of Changes in Equity, it is included in the calculation of the ending equity balances. These ending equity balances are subsequently shown on the Statement of Assets, Liabilities and Equity.

In addition, net income is the initial value reported on the Statement of Cash Flows.

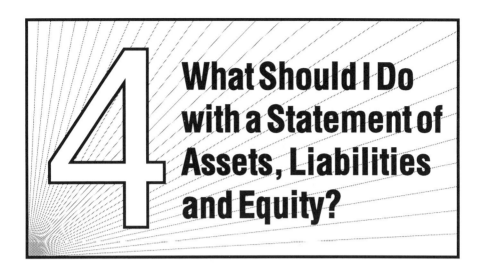

4 What Should I Do with a Statement of Assets, Liabilities and Equity?

Dr. R. M. Lave continues to review the accountant's report and financial statements for the past year. In examining the Statement of Assets, Liabilities and Equity, he wonders what to do with this information. Other than telling him how much cash he is supposed to have in the bank, and that there is a mortgage due on the building, he doesn't see any pressing need for the rest of the information that appears on this particular financial statement.

Yet, when the office manager prepares checks for him to sign, she again raises the issue of the low cash balance in their account. Dr. Lave wonders why this is so when he looks at his most recent cash balance as reported in the Statement of Assets, Liabilities and Equity, and it appears to be adequate for his immediate needs. The office manager reminds him that the balance reported on the statement was the cash balance at a specific date in time—several weeks ago. She also reminds him that the balance reported on the financial statement is not necessarily the actual bank balance at that time. Dr. Lave wonders why the financial statements should report a cash balance that is not cash available to the business!

These differences occur because of outstanding checks and because of deposits that may be recorded by the bank later than they are recorded in the accounting records. She explains that the accounting records record the checks as a reduction to the cash balance when they are written, and deposits are recorded on the day the deposit is made. However, the bank reduces the bank balance only when checks are presented for payment and records deposits made late in the day on the next business day. Thus, if there are checks that haven't been cashed or deposits that have not yet cleared, the bank balance will be different from the amount reported on the Statement of Assets, Liabilities and Equity.

Dr. Lave considers these facts and wonders whether there are other cases where the balances reported on the Statement of Assets, Liabilities and Equity don't represent the actual amount or value of the account for the business. He decides that this would be an excellent opening question for the next meeting with his accountant!

Many of the questions Dr. Lave raises should be considered by anyone who reads financial statements. This chapter will answer the questions raised above and address other related issues. Specifically, this chapter will consider:

- How are the assets, liability and equity accounts classified in the financial statements?
- How are assets, liabilities and equities valued in the financial statements?
- How do the elements of the Statement of Assets, Liabilities and Equity relate to each other and to other financial statements?
- How should you interpret a Statement of Assets, Liabilities and Equity?
- How can a physician use this information to manage a medical practice?

Before an in-depth discussion of the Statement of Assets, Liabilities and Equity occurs, it might be helpful if we review what has been written in the earlier chapters on this topic.

Overall View of the Statement

The Statement of Assets, Liabilities and Equity provides an overall view of the financial health of your medical practice at a specific point in time. Thus, remember that it should be viewed as a "snapshot," whose picture is relevant only on that particular day.

What Does It Tell You?

You should note that the title of this report describes the contents of the statement exactly; it is nothing more than a listing of assets, liabilities and equity of your medical practice. Remember that assets are the financial resources of the medical practice that are available for your use. In contrast, liabilities are the financial commitments you have made on behalf of the practice. The third component represents your ownership interest as well as the interest the practice has reinvested in itself.

One manner of determining the financial health of your practice is to focus on this statement since it reports the financial resources your practice has to work with as well as the amount of money owed by the practice. Thus, an assessment of whether or not there is enough cash available to pay the mortgage, can be determined by examining this statement.

This financial statement is commonly called the *balance sheet* for other business enterprises. It is helpful to remember that title since it reminds you that this financial statement contains a self-balancing set of information. The resources in your medical practice had to come from somewhere and there is a limited number of choices available as the source of these assets.

The first choice is for a medical practice to finance its assets by taking on a debt (e.g., obtaining a mortgage when purchasing a building). The second source of financing is through ownership contributions made by the partners. If the contribution is expected to be repaid, it would be classified as a debt similar to that of a mortgage. If, however, the contribution is considered permanent, the amount would be classified as an equity interest and would be shown in that portion of the financial statement.

The third source of financing is retained earnings. Retained earnings is often misunderstood because it is difficult to see how a practice can reinvest in itself. Assuming that the practice makes a profit, and to the extent that those profits are not actually distributed to the partners, the medical practice retains that value as an investment in itself. However, if the practice incurs a loss, the equity or ownership interest retained in the practice also goes down.

To illustrate this concept on a personal basis, assume you had an excess of your take-home pay over your monthly expenditures. If you choose not to spend the money on other items and deposit the funds in a savings account instead, you have increased your own personal equity position. If however, your expenses were more than your take-home pay, your personal equity would decline because you would have to use some of your savings to pay your bills.

The mechanics of this process for a business can be seen by tracing the flow of net income from the Statement of Revenues and Expenses, through to the Statement of Shareholders' (or Stockholders') Equity. For practices operating as a sole practitioner or as a partnership, income would flow through to the Statement of Owner's (or Partner's) Capital. These relationships were discussed in detail in Chapter 3 and illustrated in Figures 1-2 and 3-5 and it would be helpful to review these charts again.

Timing of the Statement

It is important to remember how and when the statement is prepared. This statement is dated as of the last day of the accounting period; thus, it will be dated the last day of the month, quarter, or year depending upon how often your receive your financial statements. Although it is dated as of a specific time, the actual preparation occurs several days or even weeks after that date. This is dependent on how long it takes the accounting system to process all the required transactions.

It should also be noted that although this financial statement is often the first one contained in your accountant's report, it cannot be prepared until the income or loss for the period has been calculated and processed through to the equity accounts; either retained earnings for corporations or the partner's/individual's capital account.

Now that the basics of the Statement of Assets, Liabilities and Equity have been reviewed, let's examine how the elements of the Statement of Assets, Liabilities and Equity are classified and how the value of each account is determined.

Classification of Accounts

Assets, liabilities and equity are the three components of this statement. Because there is a balancing that occurs among the three components, assets are often shown on the left, with the liabilities followed by the equity accounts shown as the balance on the right. This reporting style is called the account format and is widely used in medical practice financial statements. There is another reporting style, called the report format, which lists assets first, with the liabilities and equity accounts listed directly underneath. This reporting style is also frequently seen.

Assets

Assets are arranged in the order of liquidity, i.e., how fast can the practice convert noncash assets into cash. Thus, your first asset listed is usually cash, while the last is often some form of property and equipment. Assets are classified in this order to give any financial statement reader a quick and easy method for determining the availability of cash.

Looking at your financial statements, you may also notice additional subgroupings within the asset category, such as current assets, investments, property, and equipment, and other assets. These asset subgroupings classify your accounts by a current, versus noncurrent, status. Any asset classified as current is one that you can reasonably expect to convert to cash within one year. The assets in the other three subgroupings are considered long-term (or noncurrent) assets, whose cash convertibility is considered likely to take more than one year. It is helpful if you now examine the Statement of Assets, Liabilities and Equity for your medical practice and note the current or noncurrent status of each of your accounts.

Liabilities

Liabilities, in contrast, are arranged in the order of maturity (i.e., how fast you must repay the debt). In a manner similar to assets, liabilities are normally broken down between current and long-term amounts. Any liability on your Statement of Assets, Liabilities and Equity that is listed as current, would typically be subject to repayment within one year. Any liability listed in the long-term category does not have to be repaid until one year or after.

Equity

Equity accounts are arranged in order of permanency, with the most permanent first. Permanency is a legal concept referring to how accounts are affected in the event of bankruptcy. Thus, the stock accounts, which represent your ownership interests, are considered the most permanent and will be listed first in the equity section.

The least permanent account is the retained earnings account, which is the first account affected if the medical practice sustains a loss. Continued losses that create a negative balance in the retained earnings account, strongly indicate the ill health of a medical practice.

Valuation of Assets, Liabilities and Equity

Each financial element on the Statement of Assets, Liabilities and Equity is reported at a specific dollar value. However, how the amount is determined may be different, depending on the type of account. For example, cash is already in its cash equivalent form, so there is no need to consider the value for this account. In contrast, an asset such as property and equipment is listed at book value, determined by subtracting an accumulated usage component from the original cost of the asset. Further information on the valuation of specific accounts will be discussed shortly as each account of this statement is reviewed.

Liabilities are normally listed at the amount that would be required immediately if you wanted to pay off the debt today. This is not an area of major significance for medical practices since, other than mortgages and in some cases pension liabilities, most of the liabilities are short term and therefore, are valued at their current amounts.

In the following section, we will discuss the nature and valuation of each account on the Statement of Assets, Liabilities and Equity, using the information found on Figure 3-1 as a guide. It will also be helpful to examine your own statement in order to relate the discussion to the particular accounts which are relevant to your medical practice.

Assets

Cash

Cash is the first asset listed because it is the most liquid. A cash account for a medical practice typically consists of a petty cash fund in the office, a checking account used to pay bills, a savings account, or money market mutual funds. However, determining a value for these accounts is not necessary because they are in their cash form. In contrast, you may note an account, called marketable securities, listed on your financial statement.

Marketable Securities

In good cash management, excess available cash is transferred from a regular cash account to some type of short-term investment. This is done in order to earn a higher rate of return. The marketable securities account normally represents investments in various types of securities; money market funds, certificates of deposit, etc. Most medical practices do not have a marketable securities account. In larger medical practices with significant cash flow, however, the opportunity to maximize your rate of return by investing in short-term marketable securities should be considered.

Marketable securities were valued, until recently, at the lower of the cost on the date you invested or the current market value. However, a recent change in the accounting regulations now requires that this account be reported at the current market value as of the date of the Statement of Assets, Liabilities and Equity. Thus, to value this account, you must refer to sources, such as *The Wall Street Journal,* that will identify the market value on a particular day.

Notes Receivable

This account may arise due to the withdrawal of funds (i.e., a loan) from the practice to an individual, or because the funds are due to the practice in conjunction with a partner buy-in. Either way, this account represents an amount to be received by the practice, hence its name *notes receivable*. In some financial statements, this account may be labeled "Notes Receivable Due from Partners," while in other medical practices the notes receivable is not specific as to from whom the amount is due.

Notes receivable are valued at the amount due to your medical practice, either from a partner in your practice or from any other individual who has signed a note promising to pay a fixed amount to the medical practice.

This account may be listed as a current asset, as described in this section, but it is often listed as a long-term asset in the "Other Asset" category. Which asset category it belongs to depends upon the timing of the note. Any funds due within the immediate year are classified as a notes receivable, current; any amounts due to the practice after one year are classified as notes receivable in the Other Asset category.

Prepaid Insurance

Insurance costs are allocated over time corresponding to how long the policy is in effect. Prepaid Insurance is the unused portion of a policy that has been paid for in advance by the medical practice. For example, suppose the practice purchases a 12-month fire insurance policy for $1,200 on May 1. By December 31, eight months is "used" and four months remains as paid in advance.

Under the modified accrual basis of accounting discussed in Chapter 3, we learned that the entire amount of the policy could not be expensed in the year of purchase. Rather, a portion of the amount is expensed as time passes and the unused portion remains as an asset on your Statement of Assets, Liabilities and Equity.

This account is normally listed as a current asset because the expiration of the insurance policy is expected within one year and because cancellation of the insurance policy would normally result in a cash refund.

Prepaid Taxes

Prepaid taxes is the amount the medical practice paid in advance of when the income tax was due (i.e., quarterly estimated taxes). This account is present only for medical practices that have some form of corporate organization.

Quarterly payments are recognized as prepaid since the tax deposit was made by the practice in advance of when the final amount is due. This is done in accordance with IRS regulations that stipulate a quarterly deposit of a portion of the taxes expected to be due at year-end. This amount is listed as a current asset until year-end when it is converted into income tax expense.

Deposits

Deposits are the amounts paid by the medical practice in advance of when the goods or services are rendered. Deposits listed as current assets are expected to be returned to the medical practice within one year.

Deposits commonly occur for other items such as utility connections, or security deposits on rental property. Although these items are typically long-term in nature, they will often be classified as current due to their small dollar value.

Supplies Inventory

Office supplies inventory and medical supplies inventory are commonly found on the financial statements of a medical practice. This account is typically a current asset since the supplies are expected to be used within the next year.

These inventories are valued at whatever it costs the medical practice to purchase the supplies, including any delivery charges. Proper management of supplies inventory dictates that you make a minimum investment in this particular type of asset.

Property and Equipment

Investment in property and equipment, sometimes called fixed assets, can be substantial for a medical practice. These assets are typically classified as long-term since their expected useful life ranges from three to five years for certain types of equipment, to 30 or 40 years for the life of a building.

These assets are initially recorded at whatever it costs your practice to acquire them. However, as time passes, a portion of the cost of these assets is transferred to expense via the depreciation process detailed in Chapter 5. This process recognizes the decline in value of the asset because of time or use and occurs for all property and equipment accounts except land.

The amounts originally paid to purchase the assets are shown on the Statement of Assets, Liabilities and Equity. However, this value is then reduced by the amount of depreciation charges accumulated over time, shown in a separate account called "Accumulated Depreciation." Thus, the relevant value to consider is the *net* property and equipment (i.e., original cost less the depreciation) because it shows the value of the asset after an amount has been allocated for usage. However, land is always reported at its original cost since its value does not decrease with usage.

The common terminology for the net value reported in property and equipment is *book value*. It is important to note that book value rarely bears any relationship to the market value for these particular assets. Although it is not unusual to see a particular piece of property actually appreciating in value, most of the assets that are used by the practice decline in value over time. This decline in value corresponds to the amount of usage. Therefore, their book value, also known as depreciated value, will decline each year.

A common account found in property and equipment is leasehold improvements. Any medical practice that rents office space and spends money to renovate/decorate, will have this account. Although leasehold improvements does not represent a tangible or real asset that you actually own, it is money spent to enhance rented office space. Since there is a long-term life to the renovations, usually corresponding to the long-term life of the lease, it is treated the same way as any property and equipment.

Therefore, the value of the leasehold improvements is placed on the Statement of Assets, Liabilities and Equity and subsequently converted into expense over its useful life. The relevant time period for expensing leasehold improvements is normally dictated by the length of the lease. Thus, if you spend $20,000 renovating office space and the lease term is 10 years, $2,000 per year will be converted into operating expense each year of the 10-year life of the lease. Therefore, the book value of the improvements declines each year in the same manner as the decline in book value of property and equipment that you own.

Other Assets

This category of assets may contain a range of accounts, depending on the nature of your medical practice.

As noted in the current asset section, notes receivable which have a long-term due date, will be classified as an Other Asset. The valuation of this account is the same whether it is a short- or long-term account (i.e., it is the amount of funds due to the practice from a partner or other individual).

Goodwill is another long-term asset that may be listed in this category on the Statement of Assets, Liabilities and Equity. Goodwill is a concept that is often difficult to understand so the easiest way to describe it is to relate it to a personal situation.

Assume you wanted to purchase a home in a certain location due to the reputation of the schools in that district. You know the asking price of the house but you also know that there are several interested buyers. As a result of these factors, you offer a bid in excess of the asking price, hoping to insure the buyer's acceptance of your offer. Your willingness to pay an amount over the asking price indicates that a goodwill value for this house exists. When you actually pay the excess price, you have created goodwill.

Goodwill for a medical practice results when you pay an amount in excess of the going market price to acquire an existing medical practice. Your willingness to pay more than market value indicates that there was an intrinsic value that could not be specifically identified or attached to a particular asset of the practice. Rather, it may be the result of the reputation, name, or location of the practice, the patient list, or other items that you wish to acquire.

It is important to note that goodwill can only exist if it has been purchased in conjunction with an acquisition of another practice. Thus, you cannot simply determine that your practice's reputation has value and report goodwill in your financial reports.

Liabilities

As we discussed earlier, liabilities are arranged in the order of maturity, recognizing how quickly the debt must be paid. Those which must be repaid in less than one year are considered current; those in excess of one year are classified as long term.

Current Liabilities

NOTES PAYABLE

Notes payable, a common liability in a medical practice, is a debt that must be repaid to the holder of the note. Although a note is held by a bank, there are other types of notes payable. For example, if a partner loans money to the medical practice to cover a cash flow shortage but expects to be repaid within a year, a note payable is created and would be shown as a current liability.

The amount reported for this liability is the face value of the debt that must be repaid. Interest related to the debt is typically regarded as a separate component and is not reflected with the notes payable account.

PAYROLL TAXES WITHHELD

This liability recognizes the amount of federal, state, and local payroll taxes that you withhold from an employee's or partner's gross paycheck. This withholding is considered a liability since the funds withheld do not belong to the practice and you are responsible for ensuring that payments are promptly forwarded to the relevant taxing authorities.

This liability should not continuously grow to a significant amount on your Statement of Assets, Liabilities and Equity. If it does, it means that payments to the tax authorities are not being made. This results in substantial penalties and other problems for the medical practice and should be avoided at all costs.

ACCRUED PENSION

If your financial statement lists an accrued pension account as a current liability, it is the amount due to be deposited with the pension fund within the next year. This liability is cleared whenever deposits are made.

For practices that state that "all pension costs accrued are funded," it means that deposits to the pension fund are actually made in the same year that the expense is recorded. In this situation, an accrued pension account will not exist.

LINE OF CREDIT

As the complexity and time requirements for insurance reimbursement continue to grow, medical practices often find themselves short of cash. Until payment is received from the insurance companies, medical practices must find ways to pay their current expenses. This is often accomplished with a line of credit from a local bank.

A line of credit allows the medical practitioner to draw down funds as needed to finance the operations of the medical practice. In principle, this operates like a home equity loan (i.e., you withdraw funds at various points in time only for the amount of funds needed). With this arrangement, you pay interest only on the amount that is outstanding at any point in time.

However, there is one fundamental difference between a home equity loan and a line of credit. Home equity loans are usually used for major long-term improvements of your residence or other long-term acquisitions, such as the purchase of a car. However, a line of credit typically finances the short-term operating needs of the practice.

When you use borrowed funds for long-term capital improvements, there is a corresponding long-term benefit obtained from the use of such funds. In contrast, the medical practice often uses this debt to cover normal operating expenses. This situation should not go on indefinitely and repayments of the line of credit should be made whenever possible. Not only will this reduce the interest cost, it is a sound business practice. Thus, the line of credit should be used to cover short-term cash flow needs on an occasional basis.

INCOME TAXES PAYABLE

Income taxes payable is the amount due for federal, state, or local income taxes. This account is separate and distinct from the payroll withheld tax account, whose liability is only for payroll taxes.

Income taxes payable is the opposite of prepaid taxes, which was discussed earlier. Income taxes payable arise when it is determined that additional amounts are due to the IRS or a state/local taxing authority—that is, the amounts paid in advance are not sufficient to cover the actual amount due.

Remember that corporations are separate, taxable entities, which must recognize their own income tax impact, while partnerships and proprietorships are flow-through structures which do not have an income tax liability. Thus, whether deferred taxes or income taxes payable exist in your financial records, depends on your form of organization.

Typically, corporate income taxes are paid four times a year, 15 days after each quarter ends. Therefore, this liability should be reduced periodically.

CURRENT PORTION OF MORTGAGE PAYABLE

This liability is the total of the mortgage payments due within the next year. The rest of the mortgage payable is shown in the long-term liability section, since it represents the remaining payments due over the life of the mortgage.

It is not unusual to see the same amount in the current portion of the mortgage payable account every year since it is simply a reclassification from the long-term portion. However, you should see a yearly decline in the amount of the long-term mortgage in an amount equal to the current mortgage liability.

LONG-TERM LIABILITIES

Long-term liabilities are those due after a one-year time period. The most common long-term liabilities for a medical practice are mortgages and notes payable. Each of these accounts reports only the balance due for the years after the current year since the amount due in the upcoming year is always classified as a current liability. Thus, a long-term liability account declines each year in an amount equal to the 12 months of payments shown as a current liability.

Shareholders' Equity

Shareholders' equity, also known as stockholders' equity, shows the corporate owner-ship component of your medical practice. This section reports the balance in the common stock, additional paid-in capital and retained earnings accounts, and is reduced for stock repurchased by the medical practice. For a partnership or proprietorship, this section is simply called *capital* and reports individual capital and drawing accounts.

The common stock and additional paid-in capital accounts show what is commonly known as *contributed capital*, and the retained earnings account reports *earned capital*. Thus, the stock and paid-in capital show what the individual medical practitioners were willing to invest in the medical practice, while the retained earnings account is the amount that the medical practice reinvested in itself.

The details of the changes that occur for each of these accounts during the year are reported in the Statement of Changes in Shareholders' Equity. This statement was illustrated in Figure 3-3.

Common Stock

A common stock certificate is the vehicle used to evidence ownership by an individual in the corporation. The amount of stock certificates issued are accounted for in the common stock account. Whether the corporation is an "S" corporation or a professional corporation, the end result is the same.

Common stock usually has a par or stated value assigned when the corporation was formed. It has nothing to do with the book value of the corporation, nor does it have anything to do with the market value of the stock. Rather, it is simply a legal amount assigned to the stock.

The stock account is valued at the number of shares issued to the associates times the par value of the stock. To illustrate, if there are 1,000 shares of stock issued and the assigned par value is $5, the amount reported in the common stock account would be $5,000.

Additional Paid-In Capital

This account arises when there is a par value assigned to the common stock of the corporation **and** the value of the financial transaction is higher than the par value of the stock.

For example, assume that an associate's ownership interest is evidenced by 10,000 shares at $1 par value per share. However, the value of the buy-in was $50,000. Therefore, the effective market price is $5 per share ($50,000 ÷10,000 shares). As a result, the additional paid-in capital is the $4 difference per share between the par value ($1) and the market value ($5), times the 10,000 shares issued, or $40,000.

Retained Earnings

Throughout the earlier chapters, we have made several references to how a medical practice reinvests in itself. This reinvestment is reflected in the retained earnings account.

Retained earnings is the net accumulation of profits, losses, and payouts that a corporation makes over the life of the medical practice. Whenever profits are made, retained earnings increases; when losses occur, retained earnings decreases; and any distributions to associates also decrease this balance.

To illustrate, assume a medical practice is 10 years old. There have been seven years of profit totaling $450,000 and three years with losses of $150,000. In addition, payouts to the doctors over the 10 years totaled $90,000. As a result, the retained earnings balance would be calculated as $210,000 ($450,000 − $150,000 − $90,000).

Thus, this account represents the net result of all activities affecting the earned capital reinvested in your practice.

Treasury Stock

Whenever a medical practice repurchases existing stock from one of the associates with the intent of subsequently reissuing it to another associate at some later point in time, it is called *treasury stock*. This transaction is valued at the amount it costs the practice to acquire the shares. This value is assigned to a Treasury Stock account, where it remains until the shares are reissued. Treasury stock is shown on the statement of Assets, Liabilities and Equity as a "contra" equity account, which means that it decreases the total amount of equity invested in the practice.

Since treasury stock is a temporary reacquisition of the corporation's stock, it can subsequently be reissued to another associate. When these shares are reissued, the Treasury Stock account is eliminated. In addition, any excess amount the corporation receives over its cost of the shares, is placed in the additional paid-in capital account in the same way a new issue of stock is recorded.

For example, assume the practice purchases the shares of Associate X for $80,000, and this value is reported in the Treasury Stock account. These shares are subsequently purchased by Associate A in a buy-in transaction valued at $95,000. In this case, the Treasury Stock account would be reduced to zero and the additional paid-in capital account would increase by $15,000.

Equity Interests for Proprietorships and Partnerships

The equity section of the Statement of Assets, Liabilities and Equity examined thus far has focused on shareholder or stockholder equity. This assumed that the medical practice had a corporate form of organization. For medical practices operating as a partnership or a proprietorship, this section of the financial statement is different.

Rather than common stock, paid-in capital, and retained earnings accounts, equity is represented by individual capital accounts. The capital balance reported on the Statement of Assets, Liabilities and Equity is the balance as of the end of the year. However, the changes during the year that affect ownership transactions (i.e., profits, losses, or withdrawals from the medical practice) are shown in the Statement of Changes in Partner's or Owner's Capital, illustrated in Figure 4-1.

How Do the Financial Statement Elements on the Statement of Assets, Liabilities and Equity Relate to Each Other and to Other Financial Statements?

Relationships among the Elements

Understanding how the elements within the Statement of Assets, Liabilities and Equity relate to each other will facilitate your understanding of the financial statement. The

FIGURE 4-1
STATEMENT OF CHANGES IN PARTNER'S (OR OWNER'S) CAPITAL

	Partner A	Partner B
Balance, January 1, 1993	_____	_____
+ Net Income		
–Partner Withdrawals		
Balance, December 31, 1993	_____	_____
–Net Loss		
Balance, December 31, 1994		

relationships among the elements on this statement are centered on several key concepts, namely, (1) the source of your asset financing, (2) the parallel between current assets and current liabilities, and (3) the parallel between long-term assets and long-term liabilities.

The Statement of Assets, Liabilities and Equity tells you the source of your asset financing (i.e., how were you able to purchase your assets). Because the liabilities and equity shown on this statement are the balance to the asset side of the equation, they clearly indicate whether the assets were acquired through a debt that has to be repaid, or through equity investments in the medical practice. Knowing how the asset base is financed provides information on how much of the practice is owned outright in contrast to that which requires future cash for repayment.

Another important interrelationship is the recommended parallel between the type of asset and the corresponding liability. Classifying both assets and liabilities as current or noncurrent is not done only to indicate how fast the asset can be converted to cash, or when the debt must be repaid. They are also classified this way to allow the financial statement reader to relate current assets available to the current outstanding liabilities, and to relate long-term assets to long-term liabilities in the same manner.

Current assets should be balanced against current liabilities to determine whether there are sufficient funds available to meet the obligations. If there are not enough current funds available to pay the current debts, the practice has to consider various options, such as selling other assets to generate the needed cash. A good rule of thumb is to maintain twice as much in current assets as current liabilities. This ensures that the current liabilities can be paid promptly and that additional funds remain to apply toward payment of long-term debt.

When you initially seek financing for assets, avoid financing short-term assets with long-term liabilities. Rather, there should be a correlation between the type of asset acquired (i.e., long-term or short-term) with the financing used to obtain that particular asset. This means that you should not commit to a long-term liability for operating expenses or for assets that have a short life.

Relationship to the Other Financial Statements

The Statement of Assets, Liabilities and Equity is directly connected to two of the other financial statements. The first involves cash, where the balance reported in the Statement of Assets, Liabilities and Equity is the same amount reported as the ending cash balance on the Statement of Cash Flows. This relationship was illustrated in Figure 3-5 and it is useful to reexamine these financial statements when reading this section.

However, the relationship is more than the fact that the same number appears on two financial statements. Rather, the Statement of Cash Flows explains how your business got from its beginning cash balance to the balance that is shown at the end of the year. It does this by detailing the sources of cash inflow, as well as the uses of cash, throughout the year. Thus, when your cash balance on the Statement of Assets, Liabilities and Equity changes from one year to the next, you can easily see the details of where the cash came from and how it was spent by referring to the Statement of Cash Flows. This statement will be examined in detail in the next chapter.

There is also a direct relationship between the Statement of Assets, Liabilities and Equity and the Statement of Changes in Shareholders' Equity, which we illustrated in the prior chapter. It is the ending balances are reported on the Statement of Assets, Liabilities and Equity, but the source of the detailed information that supports the balances for these accounts can be found on the Statement of Changes in Shareholder Equity.

In summary, the Statement of Assets, Liabilities and Equity always reports totals at a point in time. To understand the details of the changes from one year to the next, you must look for the information on the two statements that show change (i.e., the Statement of Changes in Shareholder Equity and the Statement of Cash Flows).

How to Interpret Your Statement of Assets, Liabilities and Equity

There are useful standard measures available to help a financial statement reader assess a set of financial statements. These measures, known as financial ratios, have traditionally been used by analysts in examining financial statements of businesses other than medical practices. This is true for several reasons. First, medical practices typically have not been considered as a business. However, given recent changes in the health care climate, medical practices now must be evaluated in the same manner as other businesses. The second reason ratios have not been used in evaluating medical practices is because many of the ratios are not meaningful given the types of operations.

However, there are several standard ratios that can be applied to medical practices. Calculating and interpreting these measures will enhance your understanding of your own Statement of Assets, Liabilities and Equity.

Financial ratios are nothing more than relating two financial statement elements together, usually as numerator and denominator. In the next section, we will limit our discussion to those ratios which can be reasonably applied to a medical practice. The discussion will specifically focus on using standard financial ratios to perform a liquidity, financing and earnings to asset assessment.

Liquidity Assessment

A liquidity assessment answers one simple question: Can you meet your current obligations and have money left over? This is the same concept as maintaining a personal monthly budget and providing a "cushion" of cash for additional or unexpected events.

A liquidity assessment for your practice will determine how much cash or other liquid resources are available to pay off the short-term debts. This information is critical in any business but it is essential when cash flow concerns are present. Thus, using additional indicators can be helpful in assessing the liquidity status of your practice.

The quickest and easiest way to assess the liquidity of a business is to calculate a *current ratio*, which is a ratio of current assets (numerator) to the *current liabilities* (denominator). In addition, you can calculate *net working capital*, which is defined as current assets minus current liabilities. We will discuss net working capital first.

Net working capital, or current assets minus current liabilities, tells you the amount of current funds that would be available after payment of current liabilities. These available funds can then be used for other purposes, such as current period operating expenses or payments toward long-term debt. It makes good business sense to have current assets available in excess of the amounts needed to pay your current liabilities.

Net working capital answers the liquidity question in raw dollar terms. This calculation is easy to make and tells you dollars available in the short term. However, this result assumes that all the current assets are convertible to cash and are available to pay off current liabilities. This assumption has obvious limitations because a current asset, such as medical supplies inventory, may not be as liquid as a marketable security account. Therefore, you have to pay particular attention to the type of current asset available.

The second financial ratio useful in a liquidity assessment is the current ratio. This is a simple calculation where you divide current assets by current liabilities. This ratio presents the liquidity results on a relative basis. To illustrate, assume that your practice has current assets of $80,000 and current liabilities of $40,000. Your current ratio would be a 2 to 1, meaning that there are two dollars of current assets available for every dollar of current liabilities.

This ratio has the same shortcomings discussed under net working capital in that it assumes that each dollar of current assets is of equal cash value. In many medical practices, current assets are comprised of cash or cash-type assets, such as marketable securities and deposits. However, you should examine the makeup of your current assets to see how liquid they really are. Consider the following example.

CURRENT ASSETS—PRACTICE A

Cash – checking		$ 3,000
Cash – savings		10,000
Deposits		2,000
	Total	$15,000
Current Liabilities		$ 7,500

CURRENT ASSETS—PRACTICE B

Cash		$ 1,000
Advances to officers		6,000
Prepaid insurance		4,000
Prepaid federal taxes		4,000
	Total	$15,000
Current Liabilities		$ 7,500

Note that both practices have net working capital of $7,500 ($15,000 – $7,500) and a current ratio of 2:1 ($15,000/$7,500). However, it should obvious that Practice A is much more liquid than Practice B because the type of assets that they hold are quite different. Therefore, you must consider information other than pure numerical results when assessing your practice's liquidity position.

To highlight the differences in the type of current assets, you can also calculate a cash ratio. This calculation relates only the cash or cash type assets, such as marketable securities to the outstanding current liabilities. This ratio has the advantage of eliminating the noncash current assets in the assessment of liquidity.

Using the numbers from our prior example, the cash ratio readily confirms our prior assessment. Practice A's cash ratio is ($13,000/$7,500) while Practice B's ratio is ($1,000/$7,500). It is obvious that Practice B's ability to pay off its current liabilities is questionable and is a result of the type of current asset they own.

Financing Assessment

A financing assessment answers two simple questions. How are your assets financed and what is the relative balance between your debt and equity position? To illustrate, let's relate these questions to the purchase of your personal residence. In this situation, a financing assessment answers the question of whether you purchased your residence with your own funds or borrowed funds. It also defines the relationship between your borrowing and your personal contribution (e.g., you borrowed four times as much money as you personally invested).

A financing assessment for your medical practice will show how you financed the assets. However, rather than show the results in dollar terms, as illustrated on the

Statement of Assets, Liabilities and Equity, financing ratios show the information on a relative basis. The three relevant financing ratios for a medical practice are: the debt to asset ratio, the debt to equity ratio, and the short-term debt to long-term debt ratio.

The debt to asset ratio shows the percent of every asset dollar financed by debt, rather than equity. To illustrate, if your medical practice has $200,000 of debt and assets worth $1,000,000, it means that 20 percent ($200,000/$1,000,000) of your asset base is supported by debt. Therefore, the inverse is that 80 percent is financed with some form of equity, either by investor contributions or earned equity retained in the business.

Additional financial information is available with use of the debt to equity ratio. The result of dividing total debt by total equity defines the relationship between the debt and equity. Using our prior example, the $200,000 worth of debt means there was $800,000 worth of equity, since debt plus equity must equal assets ($1,000,000). Therefore, as a financing component, debt comprises only 25 percent of the equity contributions ($200,000/$800,000). This means that for each dollar of equity invested in business, there is 25 cents of debt that needs to be repaid.

The third financing consideration is the relationship between short-term debt and long-term debt. Although a business must repay both short-term and long-term debt, short-term debt requires prompt attention. Thus, if $150,000 of the $200,000 debt is short-term, it means that 75 percent of your debt financing is due within one year. Coupling the results of that information with the liquidity assessment (current ratio and net working capital) described earlier, indicates whether the medical practice should be able to meet its financial obligations.

Earnings to Assets Assessment

An earnings to assets assessment answers one simple question: Are your assets generating enough income to support the investment you made in them? On a personal level, assume your hobby was investing in the stock market and your current rate of return is 6 percent.' You decide to invest in a computer solely to more closely track your investments. If your return increases to a level that justified the investment, it was an efficient and effective purchase.

How well a business uses its assets is an important consideration. To determine how effectively and efficiently your practice uses its assets, you can calculate a ratio known as the *return on assets* ratio. This is defined as net income (from the Statement of Revenues and Expenses) divided by total assets. This calculation reduces your return on assets to a specific number. If you earn net income of $100,000 and your asset base is $1,000,000, it means your return on assets is 10 percent.

Inefficient use of assets represents lost earning power for the business. This ratio helps you to identify whether you have too high of an investment in assets over what is necessary to generate your current level of earnings. You should consider the return on assets of your business in the same way that you would consider the return on any investment. Thus, the acceptable rate of return is dependent upon a threshold that you, as a practitioner, set for the business. However, the higher the return, the better use of your assets is indicated.

Usefulness of Ratios

The ratios described above are only a small number of those widely available ratios used to assess business operations. Once again, however, we limited our discussion to those most appropriate for a medical practice.

At this point, it is important to note that a ratio, by itself, is a meaningless number. Just as you should not examine financial statements for a single year, you cannot obtain useful information by focusing on a single ratio. Thus, you should calculate ratios for a three- to five-year period, and focus on the change in the ratios over time. It will quickly help you to identify areas that need attention.

For example, assume that a medical practice makes a substantial investment in assets when the practice begins operations. In the early years, the rate of return on assets will most likely be lower than that of another practice with the same investment in assets. Logically, this occurs because the practice made a substantial asset investment prior to earning amounts that would support such an investment. As the practice grows, with a corresponding growth in earnings, the return on the assets should reach a more acceptable level.

In contrast, however, assume that the return on assets has decreased from 12 percent five years ago, to 7 percent today. It is critical to determine the cause of such a change and the two most likely causes are, either the level of investment in assets is too high, or earnings have declined. To answer the question, you need to determine whether there have been new additions to the asset base. You also need to consider your fee structure and perform an analysis of your expenses. Once you determine whether you overinvested in your assets, your fee structure has not increased in recent years, or expenses have increased, you can take appropriate corrective actions. Thus, it is important to use ratios not as an answer to a particular question, but as the question itself.

Financial analyses using ratios typically consists of two parts. The first is to examine the changes in the financial ratios and the second is to compare a company's results to published industry standards. Unfortunately, this second step of the process is not routinely performed for medical practices. Published financial statistics are available from several professional societies and some consulting groups that service medical practices. In addition comparable data from other medical practices in your area can be obtained from your accountant. Ask your accountant for data based on their client base in the medical practice field. You would then have some form of comparable results with which you can analyze your own financial data.

How to Use a Statement of Assets, Liabilities and Equity to Manage Your Medical Practice

Using the Statement of Assets, Liabilities and Equity as an aid in managing your medical practice means focusing on the information that is most relevant to your particular practice. Liquidity may be of concern for one practice while the return on assets may be the primary focus of another.

To use this information to manage your practice, you must receive your statement promptly after month end and immediately review the information with your practice's particular need in mind. Thus, you need to think about liquidity, financing, and earnings to assets and consider which of these is of critical importance at that particular point in time.

To facilitate your use of the information, examine the data using dollars and ratios. You must also put the data in perspective by considering the changes from year to year, over a three- to five-year period. Significant fluctuations in any direction require attention.

Then it is important to translate the financial information into operating decisions. For example, if you focus on the cash flow requirements necessary to pay off debt, you must answer the question of whether you have the cash available. If the answer is "no," you must consider your operating alternatives: attempt to delay the due date of the debt; try to increase cash inflows by increasing your cash collection efforts; reduce your cash outlays for other purposes; or require an equity contribution by associates with ownership status. Thus, if you allow the Statement of Assets, Liabilities and Equity to focus your perspective and then ask the right questions, the logical choices for operating decisions result.

Consider a practice whose concern centers on investment in assets. The logical question is whether the assets are appropriate for the size of the practice and are being managed properly. If the answer is "no," consider your alternatives: sell off existing assets; prohibit acquisition of new assets; or increase your net earnings by increasing revenues or decreasing expenses. Once again, using the financial statement to ask the questions benefits your practice because the operating decisions are a natural outcome of your financial assessment.

The final question that results from a focus on the Statement of Assets, Liabilities and Equity is the level of debt and whether it is appropriate for the medical practice. If the answer is "no," consider the alternatives: use existing resources to pay off debts; prohibit the acquisition of new debt; or require an equity contribution by associates with ownership status.

With the information and tools provided in this chapter, you should now be able to intelligently read and analyze your Statement of Assets, Liabilities and Equity and use the results of your analysis to make sound operating decisions.

Physician's Checklist

As a summary of this chapter, ask yourself the following questions. If you can answer "yes" to these questions, you have a good understanding of the Statement of Assets, Liabilities and Equity.

_____ 1. Do you prepare or receive a Statement of Assets, Liabilities and Shareholders' Equity on a monthly basis?

_____ 2. Do you understand why your Statement of Assets, Liabilities and Equity balances?

_____ 3. Do you know the source of your asset financing?

_____ 4. Do you know how liquid your practice is?

_____ 5. Do you know when and how frequently your debt is due?

_____ 6. Do you understand how your assets are valued?

_____ 7. Do you invest your excess cash to maximize your return?

_____ 8. Do you use your line of credit prudently?

_____ 9. Is your line of credit repaid promptly and whenever funds are available?

_____ 10. Do you understand financial statement relationships between this statement and the other financial statements?

_____ 11. Do you prepare and analyze any financial statement ratios?

Just as the Statement of Assets, Liabilities and Equity provided detailed information on the financial position of your practice, the Statement of Revenues and Expenses, as well as the Statement of Cash Flows, provide useful feedback on the operations of the practice. Chapter 5 will discuss medical practices from an operations perspective.

Questions and Answers

1. **I know the value of my building and land is worth substantially more than is reported in my Statement of Assets, Revenues and Expenses. Why?**

    The land and building recorded on your financial statements is reported at its original cost less any amount that is allocated to depreciation of the building. Thus, its value reported in your financial statement is called book value. This amount does not necessarily bear any relationship to the current value of that particular asset. Financial statements are governed by what is known as the historical cost principle. This means that amounts are recorded at the objectively determined value of the transaction, not at what an asset may sell for in the current marketplace.

2. **How are my assets, liability and equity information arranged in the financial statements?**

    Assets are arranged in the order of liquidity, that is how fast they can be converted to cash; while liabilities are arranged in order of maturity, how fast they must be repaid; and equity is arranged in the order of permanency, which is a legal concept governing the status of stock.

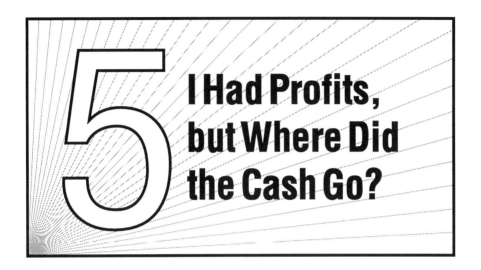

5 I Had Profits, but Where Did the Cash Go?

Dr. R. M. Lave has made tremendous progress in understanding his financial affairs. In fact, his comfort level has increased tremendously and he is now ready to tackle the two remaining financial statements, the Statement of Revenues and Expenses and the Statement of Cash Flows.

In thinking about these statements, Dr. Lave seeks the opinion of his long-time friend and colleague, Dr. Smith, who has a pediatric practice. "Which statement do you rely on to manage your practice?" Dr. Smith responds that he thinks the Statement of Revenues and Expenses is important because it tells him his revenues earned as well as his costs incurred to earn that revenue. However, he also knows that "profit" can't pay the bills and many cash transactions don't even appear on the other statements.

In contrast, the Statement of Cash Flows tells him how much cash he used to pay the bills, and what income he earned, in cash. It also tells him the other ways he obtained cash, such as his line of credit and the ways that he used cash, such as buying equipment. Since he needs cash to pay the operating costs of the practice, he examines the Statement of Cash Flows to assess his major sources and uses of cash. Without thinking about cash flow, he couldn't manage his business.

After listening to his colleague and considering which financial statement was more important, Dr. Lave realizes that it is not an either/or situation. Rather, the Statement of Revenues and Expenses and the Statement of Cash Flow complement each other and he must examine them together. However, Dr. Lave is still unsure as to which of the elements in each of the financial statements he should focus on when trying to assess his operating results.

This chapter is designed to help Dr. Lave in an assessment of his medical practice operating results. Specifically, this chapter will consider the following questions:

- How are revenues and expenses reported in the financial statements?
- How are the major sources and uses of cash identified?
- How do the Statement of Revenues and Expenses and the Statement of Cash Flows relate?
- How can you use the information from these financial statements to analyze your operating results?
- How can you manage costs in a competitive and changing environment?
- How can you improve cash flow?
- How can you utilize the information on these financial statements to manage the medical practice?

Before we begin an in-depth discussion of the Statement of Revenues and Expenses and the Statement of Cash Flows, it might be helpful to quickly review what has been written in the earlier chapters about these statements.

Overall View of the Statements

The Statement of Revenues and Expenses and the Statement of Cash Flows provide you with feedback—one on the profitability of your operation, the other on your cash flow position. Both of these statements summarize information that has occurred over a past period of time. In contrast to the Statement of Assets, Liabilities and Equity, which is a snapshot *at* a point in time, these two statements show the accumulated total of the financial transactions in your practice *throughout* a specified time period.

The Statement of Revenues and Expenses

The Statement of Revenues and Expenses is exactly as its title suggests. It focuses on transactions that directly affect profit and loss. It is nothing more than a report of the revenues and expenses of the practice over a period of time. This financial statement is commonly called the Income Statement for other business enterprises. You might also hear this statement referred to as the "P&L," which stands for profit and loss statement. This is older terminology, but it is still heard among accounting veterans who have been in practice a long time.

Regardless of what the statement is called, its objective is to report the net income for the period. Thus, it lists the revenues, subtracts the list of expenses, and produces net income. *Net* simply means after all the expenses have been accounted for, *income* with the presumption that the revenues will exceed the expenses. However, if expenses exceed revenues, a net loss is reported.

Format Flexibility

Although the Statement of Assets, Liabilities and Equity has a formalized, even rigid, structure that requires every medical practice to present their information in the same way, the Statement of Revenues and Expenses has a great deal of flexibility. In fact, there is a wide variety of presentation formats used by medical practices.

The single biggest area of flexibility is the format for reporting expenses. Some medical practices classify each element of expense as either an operating, or administrative, expense. Deciding which expense belongs in each category is normally determined by the individual practice. For example, while some practices classify telephone charges as an operating expense, others consider it an administrative expense.

In contrast, some practices simply group all expenses together, making no distinction as to the purported cause of the expense (e.g., medical operations or office administration). Others separate costs incurred by the physicians from the costs incurred by the remainder of the practice.

It is also interesting to note that the rigidity of the Statement of Assets, Liabilities and Equity with respect to the order of the accounts is not required for the Statement of Revenues and Expenses. Rather, how expenses are reported depends on the physician's, office manager's, or accountant's preference. For example, some medical practices report expenses by highest to lowest dollar value, while others report expenses in alphabetical order. There is no formal requirement in this regard. The important thing to remember is that *you* have to use the information, so structure its presentation format to facilitate *your* use and understanding.

Another common approach used by medical practices is to simply report the total operating expenses as a reduction from revenue, rather than list the details of each operating expense. If your financial statements are prepared in this way, you should also receive a supplementary schedule detailing the individual operating costs.

Of the alternatives described above, the most common approach used by medical practices is the grouping of expenses into the operating and administrative categories. Thus, it is this model that we will use in the following discussion and it is also the model that was shown in the Statement of Revenues and Expenses illustrated in Figure 3-2. Although this is the most common reporting mechanism used, remember that various practices group expenses differently.

Take a minute now to examine your own Statement of Revenues and Expenses. How are your expenses reported? Does the manner of presentation give you enough feedback on your costs? If not, perhaps you should consider changing its presentation format. We recommend that you talk to your accountant to discuss the various options available.

Timing of the Statement

The timing of the Statement of Revenues and Expenses also deserves discussion. This statement is dated for a "period ending"; thus, it will be for a period of time that ends on the last day of the month, quarter, or year, depending upon how often you prepare your financial statements. Although it is dated as of this time, the actual preparation occurs days or even weeks after that date. This depends on how long it takes the accounting system to process all of the required transactions.

Financial Statement Interrelationships

It is also important to highlight the relationship between the Statement of Revenues and Expenses and the other financial statements. If you recall our discussion in previous chapters, net income from the Statement of Revenues and Expenses is carried forward to the retained earnings account, shown on the Statement of Changes in Shareholders' Equity. This occurs because net income earned by the business represents an additional investment in the practice, unless it is distributed to the individual associates of the practice since retained earnings is one component of equity.

Thus, if the retained earnings account had a $100,000 balance before the current period income, and the Statement of Revenues and Expenses shows $15,000 in net income, the ending balance in retained earnings would be $115,000. Therefore, earnings reinvested in the medical practice increased from $100,000 to $115,000 during this time period, assuming that no distributions were made to the associates from the retained earnings account.

If distributions were to occur, they would be shown as a "drawing" for a sole practitioner or partnership form of organization, or as a reduction of retained earnings for a corporation. In any form, distribution of earnings represents a decrease in the equity in the practice.

After net income is transferred to retained earnings on the Statement of Shareholders' Equity, the retained earnings ending balance is carried forward to the Statement of Assets, Liabilities and Equity. These interrelationships were described in great detail in the earlier chapters and were illustrated in Figures 1-2 and 3-3. It might be helpful to review this information now if you are still confused about the interrelationships.

There is also a direct relationship between the Statement of Revenues and Expenses and the Statement of Cash Flows since the Statement of Cash Flows begins with net income. One of the functions of the Statement of Cash Flows is to explain the differences between the modified cash or accrual basis reporting used in determining net income on the Statement of Revenues and Expenses and the "pure" cash basis reporting used on the Statement of Cash Flows. As we did with the Statement of Revenues and Expenses, let's review what was written in the earlier chapters on the Statement of Cash Flows prior to our in-depth discussion and analysis.

Statement of Cash Flows

Once again, accountants named this financial statement in a descriptive way; it tells you how and why cash "flowed" in and out of the business.

In addition, this statement classifies each cash flow by the nature of its transaction. Thus, it tells you whether the cash transactions were caused by *operating activities* from your normal course of business, *investing activities* from your purchase or sale of assets for your business, or *financing transactions* which describe how you financially supported the medical practice.

Like the Statement of Revenues and Expenses, this statement reports activity over a period of time and therefore, is dated as of the end of the cycle, whether monthly, quarterly, or annually. As with all financial statements, it cannot be prepared until all accounting information has been processed at the end of the accounting cycle. Thus, its preparation may also take several weeks after the end of the accounting period.

In addition to the interrelationship between the Statement of Cash Flows and the Statement of Revenues and Expenses described earlier, the Statement of Cash Flows also relates to the Statement of Assets, Liabilities and Equity. The nature of this interrelationship is simple because the primary intent of the Statement of Cash Flows is to explain the difference between the cash balance shown on the Statement of Assets, Liabilities and Equity at the beginning of the year and the cash balance at the end of the year. Thus, if you want to know where your cash was spent, or why cash was received, you need to examine the Statement of Cash Flows, which gives you more details than simply the amount of the cash balance at a point in time.

Thus, the Statement of Cash Flows serves as a link among and between both the Statement of Assets, Liabilities and Equity and the Statement of Revenues and Expenses. Although a Statement of Cash Flows was illustrated in Figure 3-4, and discussed generally in this section, we will now begin our in-depth examination of both statements, beginning with the Statement of Revenues and Expenses below.

Statement of Revenues and Expenses

Revenues and expenses are the two financial components of this statement. Gross revenue for the operating period is always reported first, followed by operating and administrative expenses. Once expenses are subtracted, "Income from Operations" results. This number is important because it tells you whether you had a profit from your primary business activity.

If there are no other transactions, for example, rental revenue earned from subleasing your office space to another physician, or interest revenue earned on your investments, "Income from Operations" will be the same number as "Income before Taxes."

However, many medical practices have other types of revenues and expenses not related to their primary business purpose. These "other" revenues or expenses are called *incidental transactions* and should not be reported in the normal operating or administrative expense category. Rather, they should be shown separately so you can easily see the results of your primary operations, exclusive of these other types of activities.

Before we begin a detailed description and discussion of the Statement of Revenues and Expenses, it might be helpful to examine the format of the statement, without the detailed information shown in Figure 3-2. This will help you see how the format and flow segregate the information into its operating and incidental components (see Figure 5-1).

FIGURE 5-1
STATEMENT OF REVENUES AND EXPENSES
FOR THE MONTH ENDED 6/30/95

Revenues	From primary business activity
Less:	
Operating Expenses	From primary business activity
Administrative Expenses	
Income from Operations	Income from primary business activity
Add/Subtract:	

Other Revenues and Expenses	From Incidental transactions, such as:
	    Rental Revenues
	    Investment Revenues
	    Interest Income
	    Gain/Loss on Sale of Used Equipment

Income before Taxes	Pretax profit from all current period activity
<Income Tax Expense>	
Net Income	After tax profit from all current period activity

We will begin our discussion using the simplified illustration in Figure 5-1, focusing on the general classifications used on the statement (i.e., revenues, operating expenses, administrative expenses, and other revenues and expenses or incidental transactions). Subsequently, we will detail the individual expense accounts shown on a formal Statement of Revenues and Expenses, such as that illustrated in Figure 3-2.

Revenues

Revenues are the primary reason any business exists. For cash or modified cash basis medical practices, revenues are reported any time you receive cash for services rendered. The amount of revenues reported on the Statement of Revenues and Expenses is the sum of all amounts received for your services during the period of time identified in the heading of the financial statement.

The standard report format for revenues is a single line showing gross revenue earned for the period. It may also be identified as professional fees or income from services rendered. Occasionally, you may see a reduction from gross revenue for amounts reported as patient refunds. If you have a separate patient refund account, a subtotal for net patient revenues will be noted and this amount is the actual revenue earned for the period.

Operating Expenses

Operating expenses are those that relate to the primary and ongoing practice of medicine. Think of these costs as those that arise when you actually render medical services on a daily basis. For example, the consumption of medical supplies is directly related to seeing your patients. Likewise, wages and salaries of both the physicians and the nursing staff occur because the primary business purpose is to see and treat patients.

How expenses are classified, such as operating, as opposed to administrative, varies depending upon one's perspective. It is helpful if you examine your own financial statements and determine how your expenses are classified. For example, are they classified by operating and administrative categories? If so, which specific expenses are shown in each of these categories?

As we describe the expenses in detail in the next few pages, we will provide background information which should help you decide the appropriate classification for your expenses on the Statement of Revenues and Expenses.

Administrative Expenses

Administrative expenses are those that result from the management of a business. This is in contrast to expenses that arise from the operation of a medical practice. Another way to judge whether a cost is an administrative expense is to ask whether the expense would exist regardless of whether or not you see patients. For example, property taxes must be paid whether or not you see patients. Likewise, interest expense on a line of credit exists because you borrowed money, the result of a management decision.

Thus, these expenses typically relate to the management of office activities and are not costs that can be realistically allocated to patient services.

Other Revenues and Expenses

The "Other Revenue and Expense" category is, in some respect, a "catch-all" classification. It reports revenues and expenses that are not directly or indirectly related to your primary course of business—the rendering of medical services. Thus, any revenue or expense transaction that cannot be specifically attributable to patient care, or to the management of the practice, should be classified in this category. For example, interest earned on your bank account or investments, or renting your excess office space to another physician, is incidental to your primary business purpose.

After revenues and expenses are netted, income taxes are calculated based on the net amount if you have a corporate form of practice. After taxes are subtracted, net income results.

Now let's examine the individual expense accounts on the Statement of Revenues and Expenses, focusing on their content and the nature of the expense involved.

Detailed Expense Analysis

The following discussion examines each of the expenses commonly found on a medical practice Statement of Revenues and Expenses. We will not discuss them from the operating versus administrative classification at this time. Rather, we will focus on their nature and content as a business expense. We will describe how to report expenses according to an operating or administrative classification at the end of this section.

Wage and Salary Expense

Wage and salary expense reports the cost of employing both the physicians and the support staff, such as nurses, technicians, office manager, or receptionist. It normally includes both salaried and hourly workers, as well as part-time and full-time wages.

This is one expense account that you may see divided into several components on the financial statements. For example, some medical practices categorize wage and salary expense for the physicians as a separate component from the wage and salary expense of the office and medical support staff. Whether this expense is reported in total or segregated between the physician and support staff salaries, its content is the same. It represents the gross salaries paid to anyone who works in the medical practice.

Typically this expense category is the single biggest expense in a medical practice, constituting a significant portion of the total expenses for the practice.

Payroll Tax Expense

This account represents the employer's share of payroll taxes paid by the medical practice on behalf of each employee. The specific payroll taxes included in this account may vary according to the state and local tax structure, but you will always see the expense for social security taxes that the medical practice must contribute recorded in this account.

In a manner similar to the wage and salary account, this account may be reported for both physicians and support staff combined, or segregated into the payroll taxes for each type employee (i.e., physicians and other support staff).

This account does not include payroll taxes that are paid by the employees and withheld from their paychecks.

Medical Supplies

This account is the current period expense for supplies consumed when you render medical services. Since some practices report the drug component of medical supplies as a separate expense, medical supplies expense may or may not include drugs.

Depending on the size and type of your medical practice, medical supplies expense may also include the purchases of small medical instruments used in providing services. Small instruments are those with a useful life in excess of one year, but that have an insignificant purchase price associated with them. It is also common for medical practices to report the purchase of small instruments as a separate expense component.

Thus, medical supplies expense typically includes such things as latex gloves, cotton swabs, bandages, etc. You then need to know whether it also includes drugs given to patients or small instruments used in the medical process. Knowing how these items are recorded is important if you wish to compare your results with the results of other medical practices.

It is also important to remember that the medical supplies listed as an expense on the Statement of Revenues and Expenses are those that are actually used in the business during the current time period rather than those that are purchased. This is one area of difference with respect to cash versus modified cash basis accounting since a medical supply inventory is an asset reported on the Statement of Assets, Liabilities and Equity.

Rent Expense

Rent expense is the amount paid to rent your office facilities. It may also include rent paid to lease any operating equipment used by the practice. However, it does not include any lease payments made for rental of cars used by the physicians. This should be reported in a separate account for automobile expense.

Utility Expense

The utility expense account records the amounts incurred for all utilities, except telephone. Utilities include heat, light, water, and sewer. Typically telephone expenses are reported separately on the Statement of Revenues and Expenses.

Auto Expense

Auto expense is the amount paid to physicians for use of their personal vehicles while conducting business for the medical practice. This amount is either a flat monthly amount paid to each physician or is calculated based on actual expenses incurred. Either way, the amount paid to the physicians for any costs incurred in operating their vehicles on behalf of the business is recorded in this account.

This account may also include any rental or lease payments made by the practice for a leased car used by the physician.

Repairs and Maintenance Expense

Repair and maintenance expenses are any costs paid for the routine upkeep of your physical assets. This also includes the upkeep and maintenance of your leased assets, such as the office copier or painting the office. This account does not include such things as cleaning services that you employ.

Employee Benefits

This expense is the cost incurred for any benefits offered to your employees. Life and medical insurance premiums paid on their behalf are the most common examples of employee benefits. Some practices include pension payments in this category, while others report pension benefits separately as a pension expense.

Once again, this is a category where the employee benefits may be divided between two accounts, one for the physicians and one for the office and support staff.

Insurance Expense

Insurance expense is the payment made for insurance premiums of the medical practice. Some medical practices divide the insurance expense into its two most common components, i.e., malpractice insurance and liability insurance carried on the business.

This is one account where there may be a difference between cash basis and modified cash basis accounting and reporting. This occurs because regardless of when the premiums are paid, only 12 months of each type of insurance expense can be shown on the Statement of Revenues and Expenses.

Tax Expense

Taxes reported on the Statement of Revenues and Expense can include several types. The first is the payroll tax expense. However, this tax is typically reported in its own account as described earlier. The second tax component is property taxes, relevant only if you own your own medical office.

The third element of taxation applies only if you are a corporate form of organization and it is usually not included with the other types of taxes in this account. Rather, income tax expense is usually shown as a separate component near the bottom of the Statement of Revenues and Expenses.

Professional Dues and Subscriptions

This account records the payments made for the physicians' professional licenses and dues. These are usually paid directly to the state medical boards or medical societies to which they belong. It also includes payments made to acquire journals that are professionally related.

Note that subscriptions for magazines in the waiting room are not shown in this category. Rather, they are considered part of the cost of office supplies.

Office Supplies

This account reflects all expenses incurred to support the office and other managerial functions of the business. It includes costs for paper, pens, and folders as well as the magazine subscriptions for the waiting room noted above. It also includes such things as small calculators and any other miscellaneous expenses used by the office staff.

Professional Fees

This account includes the costs paid to your accountant for his or her consulting services and/or preparation of your financial statement information. It may also include charges for other professionals, such as legal expenses incurred by the practice or fees paid to pension consultants or other financial professionals.

Professional Meetings and Seminars

This account reports the cost of the seminars for physicians, nurses, or other support staff. In addition to the cost of the seminar, it includes transportation, lodging, and meals while attending the meeting. They are typically related to the employees' professional occupation. The bulk of this expense is usually related to the physicians but it also shows the cost of professional meetings for professional support staff.

Depreciation Expense

When property or equipment is purchased, its value is not recorded as a current period expense because there is an extended useful life associated with such an asset. Thus, it is recorded and shown as an asset on the Statement of Assets, Liabilities and Equity. When the asset is used, a portion of its cost should then be recorded as a current period expense.

Depreciation expense is the allocation of cost for use of buildings or equipment during a given time period. Depreciation is recorded in order to assign costs equal in value to its usage. This allocation must be made in order to reflect all costs incurred in generating your revenue. Without a charge to depreciation expense, the true cost of operating your medical practice is understated.

Tax Depreciation versus Financial Reporting Depreciation

The amount of depreciation calculated for tax purposes can be different from the amount recorded for financial reporting purposes. For financial reporting purposes, depreciation is often recorded using the straight line method, that is an even allocation of cost over the estimated life of the asset. For example, a $10,000 piece of equipment with a 10-year useful life will be depreciated at $1,000 per year under straight line depreciation.

However, there are also accelerated methods of depreciation used for financial reporting purposes. These methods are much like the accelerated methods of depreciation used for tax purposes where a larger amount of the cost of the asset is allocated to expense in the earlier years of the asset's life, while in the later years of the asset life, a lower amount of depreciation is recognized.

For tax purposes, depreciation is recorded using either the straight line method (same as the straight line for financial reporting purposes) or the current Modified Accelerated Cost Recovery System (MACRS). MACRS is only used for tax purposes and its application depends upon the type of asset that you acquire. Once again, you may see the same dollar figure reported for financial reporting purposes and tax reporting purposes. However, these amounts may also be different depending upon the depreciation method used.

For tax reporting purposes, there is another alternative for allocating the cost of equipment against current period income. A provision in the IRS code, known as Section 179, allows businesses to immediately charge expense for the purchase of some equipment. This immediate expense write-off reduces reported income from the business, thereby reducing income taxes. However, the real value of the asset has not declined.

Under current tax regulations, businesses are allowed to purchase equipment up to $17,500, and immediately report this purchase as an expense as long as the business reports a profit. Thus, the expense impact and income tax benefit is immediate rather than allocated over the asset's estimated useful life.

Depreciation Expense versus Cash Flow

Depreciation expense can create the single biggest difference between net income reported on the Statement of Revenues and Expenses and your operating cash flow. This occurs because cash flow is affected at the point of purchase, rather than when an asset is used, while net income is affected when the asset is used rather than when it is purchased.

Consider the following example. In 1995, your medical practice purchases a new piece of equipment for $5,000 and it is not eligible for Section 179 treatment. You expect to use the asset for five years. On a cash flow basis, there is a one-year impact only (i.e., a $5,000 outflow of cash in 1995). This information would be shown in the Statement of Cash Flows as an investing activity in that year.

In contrast, the impact of this equipment purchase on 1995's net income would be to reduce it by $1,000. In addition, 1996 through 1999 would also show a $1,000 depreciation expense, thereby reducing the net income in each of those years.

Let's further assume that your income (before depreciation) in 1995 is $100,000 and your cash flow (excluding the purchase) is also $100,000. After reflecting the depreciation expense of only $1,000, net income would be $99,000. However, since you spent $5,000 of cash, your cash flow will not match your expense recognition in the same period and cash flow is reduced to $95,000. That is why you can have profits of one value but have a different amount of cash.

Interest Expense

Interest expense is the charge paid to a bank or other creditor for the use of borrowed money. The more significant the debt of your practice, the larger the interest expense on the Statement of Revenues and Expenses.

Now that we have examined the elements of expenses in the medical practice, the next logical step is to analyze those costs. In order to do so, we must examine the nature of costs and how they respond to changes in your operating policies and procedures. To perform this cost analysis, we will consider expenses from several perspectives. After the analysis, we will reexamine the Statement of Revenues and Expenses and show you how you can interpret it as an aid in managing your medical practice.

Cost Analysis

The expenses listed on your financial statement are the total operating costs for your medical practice in a given time period. Although each account has its own particular characteristics described earlier, expenses must be regrouped in various ways in order to assess your costs and their corresponding change to your management decisions. We will discuss three ways to group expenses.

Fixed, Variable, and Semivariable Costs

The first way to group expenses is by fixed, variable, and semivariable costs. We briefly introduced this concept of cost analysis in Chapter 3, when we discussed financial statement results in an introductory manner. Understanding the nature of costs and how they change with changes in patient volume, operating hours of the medical practice, the addition or deletion of services, or office locations is critical. The subsequent analysis is meaningful only if you know how specific costs relate to their underlying activity.

To begin, you must remember the definitions of fixed, variable, and semivariable costs. Variable costs are those that increase or decrease whenever there is an increase or decrease in the number of patients that you see. For example, medical supplies used will increase if you see five more patients today than you did yesterday. Likewise, if you see 10 fewer patients the amount of medical supplies would also decline.

In contrast, fixed costs are those that do not change when there is an underlying change in the volume of patients. For example, depreciation expense does not depend on the volume of patients you see. Likewise, rent expense paid for office facilities does not increase or decrease with a change in the number of patients you see. An easy way to remember fixed costs is: even if you did not see any patients, the cost would exist.

Semivariable costs have some of the characteristics of both fixed and variable costs. These costs change with the volume of patients seen but not in the direct way that variable costs change. Rather, semivariable costs typically increase in a "step" fashion (see Figure 5-2). For example, the number of nurses or technicians used in the practice will increase only at certain stress points. When the volume of patients increases to a certain level, you will add the necessary staff to treat the patients.

To illustrate, one nurse may be able to process from 1 to 12 patients per hour, thus your costs remain at a certain level for patients 1 through 12. Once the thirteenth patient is added, you need more staff. Nurse two would be able to see patients 13 through 24 at which point a third nurse is needed. Thus, staff cost increases with the volume of patients, but in intervals other than a direct one-on-one increase.

Thus, whenever you make management decisions that have cost implications, you must consider how costs will react to that change. How costs react depends upon the type of costs: fixed costs remain unchanged (unless you invest in a new office location); variable costs change on a direct proportionate basis; and semivariable costs increase in ranges.

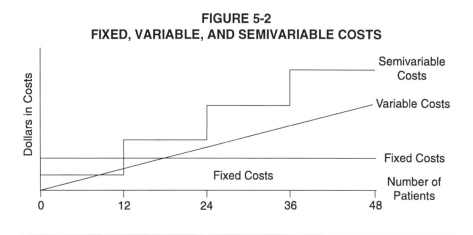

FIGURE 5-2
FIXED, VARIABLE, AND SEMIVARIABLE COSTS

Direct versus Indirect Costs

Examining expense components from a direct, versus an indirect, basis is another way to analyze your costs. This analysis is also beneficial in anticipating the reaction of costs whenever business decisions are made.

Direct costs are those that are clearly and definitively associated with rendering patient services. Nurses working in the practice, medical supplies used, and your medical malpractice insurance are all examples of direct costs incurred to meet the needs of patient treatment. In other words, these costs would not be incurred if you were not in the business of providing medical services to your patients.

Indirect costs are those incidental or nonrelated to the direct function of treating patients, or are those which have no reasonable basis for assigning costs to patients' care. For example, utilities, auto expense, or professional dues and subscriptions are indirect costs. Although these costs are necessary business expenses, they could not reasonably be allocated as costs incurred for the direct welfare of the patient.

Notice how the breakdown of direct versus indirect costs is similar to our earlier discussion on the classification of operating versus administrative expenses. Therefore, to determine how various costs should be classified for reporting on the Statement of Revenues and Expenses, ask yourself whether they are direct or indirect costs, relative to your business purpose of providing medical services to patients.

Material, Labor, and Overhead

A third method of examining your cost components is to classify each expenditure by materials used in patient treatment, labor charges paid, and overhead items, such as utilities. Categorizing your costs by material, labor, and overhead components is helpful if you want to determine the total cost of performing a particular procedure.

We recognize that costing your "product" (i.e., the services you render in treating patients) has not characteristically been done in the past. However, this concept is being used with increasing regularity today, particularly in cost accounting for hospital and health maintenance organizations and can easily be applied to your medical practice. Examining your costs from this perspective helps you to determine whether the fees charged for a given procedure actually cover all of your costs incurred in rendering services.

Is Cost Analysis Necessary?

You may wonder about the wisdom or necessity of evaluating your costs from the three perspectives noted above (i.e., fixed, variable, and semivariable; direct and indirect; and material, labor, and overhead components). Given the tough competitive environment physicians now face, understanding your cost components helps you in evaluating the results of your managerial decisions. Essentially you need to know: how costs are affected by changes in operating policy; what it costs you to provide a given service; and which costs can be allocated directly to patient care, in contrast to those that are managerial in nature. Performing these cost analyses helps you evaluate the results of your decisions.

You can use this information in combination with the concept of marginal costs. Marginal cost is the next dollar spent to generate one additional dollar in professional fees. Such an analysis will also help you determine answers to such questions as: Should I offer additional office hours; should I seek additional office locations; or can I reduce my staff size?

Cost accounting and economic concepts dictate that you should seek a situation where your marginal cost equals marginal revenue. At first this sounds as though you won't make a profit since marginal profit would be zero. However, in fact, you will be maximizing your profit since you will be taking advantage of every opportunity for profits to exceed costs.

For example, in evaluating whether you should add office hours, you must perform two steps. First, identify what additional costs would be incurred. This can be answered with the cost analyses identified above. Second, calculate whether the marginal revenues will equal or exceed the marginal costs. If marginal revenues do not at least equal the marginal costs, it doesn't make good economic sense to offer additional office hours.

This is not to say that hours should not be added from a medical practice development or patient treatment perspective. Rather, it is simply the first step of a cost and economic analysis. It may very well be that these other factors have a more significant impact on your operating decisions. Although this may be the case, you must also understand the financial impact of those decisions. Thus, consideration of each of your cost components, comprehension of how they change with changes in your current operations, and evaluation of the end result of those decisions, all require that you understand the nature of costs, and perform the cost analysis, described in this section.

Interpreting Your Operating Results

In Chapters 3 and 4, we introduced the concept of interpreting financial statement results through the use of additional analysis tools, such as common-sizing, trend analysis, and ratio calculations. We will now consider their use in the analysis of a Statement of Revenues and Expenses.

Common-Sizing

Common-sizing your Statement of Revenues and Expenses is the easiest place to begin your analysis. Unlike the Statement of Assets, Liabilities and Equity, which typically has no common-size information presented by your accountant, the Statement of Revenues and Expenses normally has prepared this information for you.

Common-sizing the Statement of Revenues and Expenses includes each expense component as a percentage of the professional fees earned in the same time period. This restates each financial statement element on a relative basis, using revenue as the common denominator. Its results show the relative importance of a particular expense component. For example, wages and salaries might be 40 percent of fees while medical supplies are only 4 percent.

This type of information is particularly important for operating decisions. Understanding the nature of costs described earlier, in conjunction with common-size financial statement information, shows you the significance or importance of one particular item. Therefore, if you want to change one aspect of the practice and the expected increase will affect one of the significant costs identified with common-sized information, you must closely monitor the effects of the decision.

However, if the incremental costs incurred are "immaterial" in nature (e.g., they represent 1 percent of your revenues), you would not need to spend a great deal of time contemplating the decision. Thus, common-sizing your Statement of Revenues and Expenses helps you to prioritize the importance of a particular cost element.

Another way you can determine the significance of a particular operating cost is to common-size the expense component as a percentage of total operating costs. This gives you an additional perspective for evaluating the importance of a particular cost component. When you are trying to make decisions that will change your costs, it might be helpful to know that your wage and salary costs are 70 percent of your operating costs, in addition to knowing that they are 45 percent of gross revenues. Thus, restating cost components as a percentage of total costs highlights the significance of one particular cost, relative to the other operating costs of the practice.

Trend Analysis

In Chapter 4, we also introduced the concept of trend analysis. Trend analysis looks at the changes in your operating results over time. Trend analysis can be performed using dollars or the change can be put on a relative basis by calculating the dollar change in an account from one period, and dividing the result over the earlier time value. Trend analysis is normally prepared for a three- to five-year time period.

What trend analysis helps you to identify are the significant changes in a particular revenue or expense component. It is important to remember, however, that it does not explain the changes. Rather, it simply points you in the right direction so that you can ask the relevant questions and determine why the changes occurred. Thus, trend analysis does not answer your questions, it simply asks the questions. *You* must find the answers to the questions and then translate them into operating decisions.

To illustrate trend analysis, assume professional fees were $100,000, $120,000, $140,000, $80,000, and $130,000 in years one through five. Calculating the change on a percentage basis highlights the obviously significant decline in year four. The percentage changes are: 20 percent increase from year one to year two, 17 percent increase from year two to three, a 43 percent decrease from year three to year four, and a 62½ percent increase from year four to five. Obviously, years three through five indicate a major change in the practice, such as one associate leaving in year four and being replaced in year five.

Removing that isolated factor (i.e., excluding year four) still indicates a slow but steady decline in the growth pattern of fees earned. Once you determine this, you must identify its reasons. Some potential explanations: lower number of patients; a change in the type of services provided (e.g., dropping the OB part of an OB-GYN practice); cash collections from patients and insurance companies declined; or a new medical practice introduced stiff competition.

Once you determine the course of the change, you can then decide how to react to the change. Trend analysis should be performed on any significant financial statement element, that is identified as a result of the common-sizing of the Statement of Revenues and Expenses described earlier. Thus, common-sizing and trend analysis go hand in hand.

Ratio Analysis

The concept of ratio analysis was introduced in Chapter 4 as a standard financial statement analysis tool used to assess the financial results of a business. In Chapter 4, we noted that ratios have not traditionally been calculated by medical practices. However, there are several standard ratios that are relevant to your medical practice.

Remember that financial ratios relate two financial statement elements together, expressed as a numerator and denominator. Their advantage is that they reduce financial statement values and relationships to a single number. However, you must also remember the caution that we mentioned in Chapter 4, concerning their usefulness. Ratios by themselves are meaningless. Just as you cannot use financial statements prepared for a single year in your decisions, the usefulness of a single ratio is questionable. Thus, you need to calculate ratios for a three- to five-year period, and more importantly, focus on the change in the ratios over time. This helps you quickly identify areas that need your attention.

As we indicated in our discussion of trend analysis, performing a ratio analysis does not answer questions. Rather, ratios highlight your need to assess a particular component, or change, that occurred in your practice. Once you have identified the cause(s) of the change(s), you can then translate your assessment into operating decisions. Finally, your ratios might be compared to ratios for other medical practices.

Although standard industry information is not widely available, certain operating statistics are published by various medical associations and consulting firms who specialize in medical practices. In addition, standard industry ratios for medical practices in your area may be available from your accountant if they service a large number of health care professionals. This gives you a comparison base in your geographical area.

To summarize, performing a financial ratio analysis requires four steps: first, calculate the ratio; second, examine the changes from period to period; third, identify the cause of the change; and fourth, compare your information to the ratio results of other medical practices.

The financial statement ratios relevant for the analysis of your Statement of Revenues and Expenses, are those that are characteristically referred to as *profitability ratios*. There are four relevant ratios in this category: the operating expense percentage; the income from operations percentage; the net income percentage; and the administrative expense percentage.

Operating Expense Percentage

The operating expense percentage is calculated by dividing total operating expense by total professional fees earned. This ratio tells you what amount of fees are consumed by operating costs. It also tells you whether your practice can control those costs by evaluating any increase in operating expenses relative to any increase in fees earned.

To illustrate, assume in year 10 that your medical practice had $200,000 of professional fees earned and $140,000 in operating expenses. Therefore, your operating expense percentage is 70 percent (140,000/200,000). Comparing this result to years eight and nine, when the ratio was 60 and 62 percent respectively, indicates that you are not controlling your costs as well as in the past years.

The primary benefit of this ratio is the ease with which it can be calculated, particularly for medical practices who report their current period expenses divided into operating and administrative expense categories. If your financial statements do not segregate current period expenses into these categories, an additional breakdown is required to calculate this ratio.

Income from Operations Percentage

The income from operations percentage is calculated by dividing income from operations (income after your operating and administrative expenses) by total professional fees earned. This ratio indicates your medical practice's ability to generate income from your primary business purpose. This result should be examined in conjunction with cash flow from operations, discussed later in this chapter.

Net Income Percentage

The net income percentage is calculated by dividing net income by total professional fees earned. This ratio simply states your net earnings on a percentage basis rather than on a dollar basis.

For example, if your medical practice generated $500,000 worth of professional fees and net income of $25,000, it earns a net profit of 5 percent, or five cents on every dollar of professional fees earned.

This ratio is easy to calculate and is a succinct measure of your medical practice's current period results.

Administrative Expense Percentage

The administrative expense percentage is the corollary to the operating percentage and is calculated by dividing total administrative expenses by professional fees earned. This ratio indicates the amount of your professional fees consumed by administrative expenses.

Obviously, the operating expense percentage should be higher than the administrative expense component. If it is not, either the classification of operating expenses is incorrect or you have too much invested in the managerial support function of your medical practice.

As a final note, remember that calculation and examination of a single ratio is worthless. However, evaluating your financial results by examining the change in ratios over time, provides you with useful information for managerial decision making.

The Statement of Cash Flows

The Statement of Cash Flows is relatively new compared to the other financial statements. In fact, it was not required for businesses until the late 1980s. Although many medical practices do not receive this statement, it provides critical operating information for your business. As the need for good cash flow management continues to increase for medical practitioners, this statement will continue to increase in importance.

The Statement of Cash Flows summarizes your cash transactions for the year. All cash inflows and all cash outflows are shown separately on the statement so you can see both the sources of your cash and where cash is spent.

This statement also provides the details that explain the change from one year to the next in the cash balance reported on the Statement of Assets, Liabilities and Equity. Without the cash flow information, you can only determine that your cash balance increased or decreased, but you won't know the reasons for the change.

Not only does the Statement of Cash Flows tell you sources of cash and how cash is spent, it also groups the cash inflows and outflows by type of activity. Thus, every cash flow is classified as either an operating, investing, or financing activity. These classifications are useful in evaluating the financial strengths or weaknesses of your practice. Using this information to interpret the Statement of Cash Flows will be discussed.

Operating Activity

The operating activity portion of the Statement of Cash Flows is listed first and is the most useful because it tells you how much cash was generated from your primary business purpose (i.e., treating patients). If you are earning revenues and collecting cash, incurring expenses and paying cash, the only difference between net income and net cash flow from operations should be for noncash expenses, such as depreciation or allocation of medical supplies inventory to expense.

Because the operating activity section tells you the amount of cash flows resulting from your primary business operations, you should examine this section to determine if your practice generates enough cash from its primary purpose to support a business. Although this may not always happen, a chronic shortage of cash generated from operations tells you that you will not remain a viable entity without a cash infusion from other sources.

Investing Activities

The cash inflows and cash outflows detailed in the investing activity section highlight the results of your "investment" decisions. Investment decisions in this sense refer to your purchase of equipment or other long-term assets for the business. Even if you decide to invest in securities to maximize interest earned on unneeded cash, the investment is also reported in this section.

Investment in assets used by the practice or investment in securities to earn interest on excess cash are two very different investment alternatives. For the overall health of the medical practice, you must invest in the assets needed for operating the business before you invest in other types of assets not related to your primary business purpose.

The investment decisions described above (i.e., the purchase of business assets), result in an outflow of cash. In contrast, cash inflows are generated when you sell assets of the business. To illustrate, if you sell equipment that you no longer use or sell the securities because you now need the cash, a cash inflow to your business results. If there are more cash inflows than outflows in the investing section, you are actually selling a part of the asset base of the company. In contrast, more cash outflows than inflows result from your cash investment in the asset base of the practice.

Financing Activities

Cash inflows from financing activities occur when you borrow money or obtain equity contributions from the associates of the practice. Cash outflows from financing activities result when you repay debt, repurchase the stock of an associate, or make distributions to the ownership interests in the practice.

The financing information shown on the Statement of Cash Flows, coupled with the debt and equity assessment described in Chapter 4, helps you to assess the level of debt and equity appropriate to your practice.

You should also note that it is possible to have noncash transactions in the business that would not be seen on any part of the statement. For example, the purchase of equipment totally on credit would not be shown. Rather, when you repaid the debt, the cash payments would be classified as a financing activity.

Now that you understand the basic fundamentals of the Statement of Cash Flows, let's evaluate its results.

Interpreting the Statement of Cash Flows

The Statement of Cash Flows is unique because it is the only statement that is prepared on a total cash basis. In other words, there is nothing reported on this statement that did not go through your cash account.

This statement is also unique because there is no financial ratio, trend analysis, or common-sizing that can be used to help you interpret the results. You may wonder how the statement is useful if there are no additional procedures or calculations that can be used to help with its interpretation. Simply, there are several key concepts that make this statement useful. Master these concepts and the statement is useful for analyzing your business results.

To begin, you must disregard the myth that only cash inflows are good. Cash inflows are beneficial in certain circumstances but not in others, depending on the underlying event. For example, assume that cash generated from operations was $10,000, cash generated from financing activities was $50,000, while cash outflows from investing activities of $25,000 were noted. You should not conclude that cash inflows from operating and financing activities were good, nor assume that it is a negative situation when investing activities use more cash than they generate. For an explanation, read on.

Interpreting Operations

The single best indicator of whether or not your practice is supporting itself is to see if you generated cash flow from operations. If there is no cash flow, or negative flow generated from operating activity, it means that you had to finance your current period activity with debt or equity rather than through current earnings. Although this may occur occasionally, it should not happen frequently or consistently. Without the ability to generate cash from your operations, you are doomed to fail.

You must also examine the related financial elements within and among the financial statements. To illustrate, assume that your practice had a profit of $40,000, but your cash balance declined from $30,000 last year to $10,000 this year. Once again, these results highlight the difference between net income and cash flow. Net income is the difference between revenues and expenses calculated on a modified cash basis, while cash flows are calculated on a strict cash basis. Therefore, the fact that you had profits, but your cash balance declined, should not be considered unusual.

When analyzing and interpreting the Statement of Cash Flows, you must always begin with the question: Did operations contribute to the cash of my business? If the answer is "no," you have problems to address. If the answer is "yes," you want to determine whether the volume of cash generated from operations was sufficient. To do this, you must evaluate your cash flow needs. This information can be found in the financing and investing portions of the statement.

Interpreting Financing Activity

The financing section of the Statement of Cash Flows tells you how your practice depended upon debt. If there is more cash inflow than outflow in this section, it means that you borrowed more money than you repaid or you had physicians contribute additional equity money. In contrast, a net cash outflow means that you paid off more than you borrowed in the current time period or you repurchased stock of an associate in excess of the buy-in of stock by another physician. Which situation is appropriate for your practice is something you need to determine.

This assessment needs to be made while examining your cash flows from operations. If there is not enough cash generated from operations, you may have no choice but to borrow additional funds or seek more equity contributions from your associates. These funds will then be shown as a cash inflow.

However, if you generate cash from operations, you will not have to borrow and you can use the cash to repay debt. This decision results in more cash outflows than cash inflows from financing activities. Therefore, even though you had cash outflows which exceeded cash inflows, it actually indicates a strong financial position for your practice since you paid off more debt than you acquired.

Interpreting Investment Activity

Last, but not least, you must consider the investment section of the Statement of Cash Flows. This is also a section where it may be beneficial to see more cash outflows than inflows because it means you are consistently reinvesting in the practice. This reinvestment has a long-term benefit. Although it may require significant cash outflows today, investment in the business through purchase of such items as property and equipment yields long-term benefits.

The Statement of Cash Flows has an inherent limitation—it reports on past cash flow activity. However, you need to budget and manage cash flow today and in the future, not solely dwell on past information. To plan for your practice's cash needs, you need to consider operating policies that will help you maximize your cash flow position.

Increase Your Cash Flow

Cash flow can be managed best by employing two tactics: (1) delay all cash payments until necessary and (2) collect and process cash due to the practice as quickly as possible. It should be obvious that you have more control over cash payments than you do over cash collections, but both require your attention. Therefore, consider the following recommendations:

Cash Payments

1. *Pay* all bills *on the due date* or the last day that a worthwhile discount is available. *Do not pay* your suppliers or creditors *early.* Why help their cash flow position when you have your own to worry about?

2. Budget your immediate future cash needs on a monthly basis. This is particularly critical in the early months of the year before patients meet their deductibles.

3. Use your line of credit only when absolutely necessary and only at the point in time when you know the specific amount needed. Don't draw down "rounded" amounts; if you need $1,800 to meet your payroll this week, don't draw down $2,000.

4. Take advantage of all worthwhile discounts offered by your suppliers. A 2 percent discount for 20 days translates into 36 percent annual interest rate.

5. Use the least cost option for available credit. Although your equipment suppliers may offer extended credit terms, chances are that their interest cost will well exceed that of your line of credit.

Cash Receipts

1. Insist on payment at the point of service.

2. Assign the responsibility for collection follow-up to an individual who can produce results.

3. Ask for a daily report of collection activity.

4. Send monthly statements to your patients and phone the patient shortly after the mailing to ask when the payment will be made.

5. Be flexible but try to obtain a commitment for a portion, if not all, of the amount due.

6. Process and deposit cash daily.

7. File for insurance reimbursements immediately.

8. Apply your collection practices to both insurance companies and patients.

We readily recognize that you can control your cash disbursements but that cash receipts are a function of a wide variety of events, most of which are beyond your control. However, this simply means that you must be extremely smart in managing your payments to others while you await payment from patients and insurance carriers. Many of the recommendations listed above will improve your cash flow position by tightening your policies and procedures over cash disbursements while encouraging prompt collection of receipts.

How to Use Financial Information to Manage Your Medical Practice

Throughout this chapter, we have tried to illustrate the integral nature of expenses and cost flow analysis, as well as cash flow and cash flow analysis, and their impact on your business decision making. In essence, analyzing your financial results tells you how your medical practice is functioning with the current operating policies and procedures in effect.

The most valuable piece of information you should remember from this chapter is to always measure the effect of your operating decisions. Only then will you be able to assess the results of your decision making. However, to measure their effect, you need to thoroughly understand the nature of income determination, cash flow, and cost assessments.

Physician's Checklist

As a summary of this chapter, ask yourself the following questions. If you can answer "yes" to these questions, you have a good understanding of the Statement of Revenues and Expenses, the Statement of Cash Flows, cost analysis, and their usefulness in providing feedback on your business.

_____ 1. Do you understand the fundamental differences between net income and cash flow?

_____ 2. Do you understand the financial statement interrelationship between the Statement of Revenues and Expenses and the Statement of Cash Flows?

_____ 3. Do you understand the difference between primary business activity and incidental business transactions, such as rental revenues?

_____ 4. Do you understand the different classification of operating and administrative expense?

_____ 5. Do you understand the content of each of your expense accounts?

_____ 6. Do you understand the difference between depreciation expense for tax purposes and depreciation expense for financial reporting purposes?

_____ 7. Do you understand the difference between operating, financing, and investing activities as shown on the Statement of Cash Flows?

_____ 8. Do you understand why not all cash outflows are bad?

_____ 9. Do you understand the distinction between fixed, variable, and semivariable costs?

_____ 10. Do you understand direct versus indirect costs?

_____ 11. Do you prepare financial statement ratios and use them to help you in the analysis of your Statement of Revenues and Expenses?

Now that we have examined the operating aspects of your daily activity, we have finished our review of the financial statements you receive from your accountant. However, financial statements alone do not include all of the necessary and relevant information needed to have a thorough understanding of your medical practice results.

Therefore, we have included Chapter 6 on the footnote disclosures that accompany your financial statements. This information is designed to help you interpret your financial statement footnotes, as a basis for a more in-depth financial and operating analysis of your practice.

Questions and Answers

1. Why aren't net income and cash flow equal?

Net income and cash flow aren't equal because the net income includes noncash items, such as depreciation. In contrast, cash flow is determined through actual cash receipts and cash disbursements by the medical practice.

2. How can I increase my cash flow?

You can increase your cash flow by taking measures to speed the collection process, and delaying your payments as long as possible. Some examples include: depositing cash daily, utilizing aggressive collection policies and procedures, only paying bills on the actual due date, taking advantage of all available discounts, and budgeting your cash flow needs on a monthly basis.

3. How can I project changes in operating costs if I decide to increase my office hours or add an additional office location?

In order to understand how costs react to your management decisions, you must understand the fundamental nature of costs. There are three types of costs: fixed costs, semivariable costs, and variable costs. Fixed costs are those that will not change as your level of output or use changes. For example, seeing more patients in a given day does not change the depreciation costs associated with owning your building, or your cost of a fixed rental contract. In contrast, variable costs change directly with changes in the level of use (volume). For example, medical supplies used increase your costs for every patient that you see.

In between fixed and variable costs are semivariable costs. These costs change, but not on a direct level with output. Semivariable costs have some of the characteristics of fixed costs and some of the characteristics of variable costs.

4. Why isn't tax depreciation the same as depreciation for financial reporting purposes?

Tax depreciation methods are determined by the Internal Revenue Service, while depreciation methods used for financial reporting purposes are determined by generally accepted accounting principles. Thus, there are two different regulatory groups that determine methods used for depreciation.

6

Explain the Notes to the Financial Statements in English, Please!

Dr. R. M. Lave now feels quite comfortable with his financial affairs. He has mastered the language of accounting and finance. He understands why his practice is organized as a professional corporation and he knows how to analyze the information contained in his monthly and quarterly financial statements.

As he sips his coffee and contemplates his daily schedule, one question remains. In the accountant's annual report, he sees a section entitled "Notes to the Financial Statements" that appears at the end of the financial statements. As he begins to read this material, he has many questions.

Dr. Lave recalls that during his academic training as a medical student, footnotes were something that could often be skipped because they usually contained unimportant detail that only needed to be read if the reader was especially interested in a specific point. However, as he skimmed the financial footnotes, he saw that they mentioned some important events peculiar to his business.

As a result, he wonders why these notes appear only in the annual report received from the accountant, rather than with the monthly and quarterly reports. He also wants to know how the notes to the financial statements relate to the other information in the financial statements, and to the accountant's report? Above all, he wants to know what to do with the difficult, and often detailed, information contained in these notes?

Dr. Lave's questions are not unusual. In fact, many financial statement readers do not understand the note disclosures and as a result give cursory, if any, attention to them. However, these notes, often referred to as footnote disclosures, or just footnotes, will enhance Dr. Lave's understanding of his financial condition and operating results.

This chapter will address the issues that concern Dr. Lave. Specifically, it will answer the following questions:

- What is the purpose of notes to the financial statements?
- What information do they provide?
- How does the information in the note disclosures relate to the numerical results presented in the financial statements?
- How is footnote information useful for managing the medical practice?

The Basics of Note Disclosures

The notes to the financial statements are a critical part of your financial statement package. The amount and type of data they present are designed to add to your level of knowledge of the financial aspects of your business. This, in turn, should enhance your understanding of the financial condition of your medical practice. Consequently, proper use of this information will help you manage all aspects of your operations.

We readily admit that reading the note disclosures is a tedious process and, rather than clearly answering questions, they may actually confuse you. As a result, there is a tendency for you and other financial statement readers to overlook, or even disregard, the note disclosures. We caution you not to ignore this information. If you want to completely understand your financial affairs, you must analyze the numerical data from the financial statements in conjunction with any footnote information provided.

As you glance at your financial reporting package, you will see that the notes to the financial statements are mostly narrative in nature. They are presented in this way because note disclosures are designed to supplement the numerical information presented in the financial statements. Another purpose of the narrative is to provide background information for interpreting your financial results. Thus, notes are critical because they give you additional information that may not, or cannot, be presented as a number in the financial statements.

Reference to the note disclosures usually appears in the first paragraph of the accountant's report, where it refers to supplementary information presented in conjunction with the financial results. However, the accountant's report may also contain a statement concerning the omission of supplementary disclosures. It is not uncommon for the notes to be omitted in monthly or quarterly financial reporting. The decision to omit this information rests with you, the physician. However, note disclosures are normally presented with year-end financial statements.

You may wonder why footnotes are considered necessary, if they can be excluded in monthly and quarterly financial reporting. Perhaps the answer to that question will be clearer after we examine the specific information contained in the individual note disclosures later in the chapter. The important thing to remember is: if the lack of information hampers your ability to understand your financial results, then note disclosures should be included in your monthly, quarterly, and annual financial reports.

It is also important to realize that the lack of note disclosures can affect the interpretation of, or conclusions by, other financial statement readers. Thus, if several people receive your financial statements, the note disclosures should be included in order to provide complete information. If, for example, you are the only reader of the financial statements, you are a solo practitioner and do not need to provide financial information to a bank or other creditor, omitting note disclosures is not usually a problem.

However, we do not recommend that you omit note disclosures if there are multiple physicians in the practice or if the financial statements are to be used by others outside of the medical practice. For example, if the medical practice applies for a mortgage in conjunction with the purchase of a building, the financial statements containing the note disclosures should be given to the bank.

Specific Note Disclosures

Let's assume, for the sake of the following discussion, that you have decided to omit the note disclosures in your monthly and quarterly financial reporting. Subject to the limitations discussed above, this is not a problem. Thus, our discussion in the next several pages will focus on the notes found most often in your year-end financial reports.

Take a minute now to refer to a copy of your most recent annual report and read the information contained in your note disclosures. Some of the notes probably won't make a lot of sense to you, but don't despair. After reading the next several pages of this chapter, you should have a better understanding of what the information contained in these notes actually means.

Note disclosures typically begin with an overall or capstone note called, "Summary of Significant Accounting Policies." This particular note contains a great deal of information on the "how" and "why" of your accounting and financial reporting. This note typically includes information on the basis of accounting used by the practice (e.g., cash or modified cash—see Chapter 3); relevant information on the form of organization (e.g., proprietorship or corporation—see Chapter 2); how your property and equipment are depreciated (e.g., straight-line or accelerated methods—see Chapter 5); and so on.

While the note disclosures for every medical practice contain this first capstone note, the remaining notes vary depending upon the type of medical practice, the size of the operation, and the complexity of your financial transactions. In the following pages, we will describe the type of information you should find in your note disclosures and we will help you interpret what the note actually means. We readily recognize that interpreting the information contained in the notes is difficult. Therefore, we recommend that during this discussion, you frequently reread your practice's notes to see if they become clearer. Hopefully, relating the information from your own practice to this discussion will facilitate your understanding.

Our discussion will begin with the information contained in the first footnote (i.e., the Summary of Significant Accounting Policies). We will then highlight and discuss the notes found most frequently in the financial statements of a medical practice. A topical summary of the information that appears most frequently in the notes to the financial statements can be found in Figure 6-4. It will be helpful if you periodically refer to this summary while you are reading the chapter.

Summary of Significant Accounting Policies

The first note to any financial statement package is the Summary of Significant Accounting Policies. This note tells you what specific accounting policies and procedures are used by your particular practice. This note is necessary because there are different methods of accounting that are allowed under generally accepted accounting principles. Therefore, the accounting methods used by a specific practice must be identified so that readers have complete information to interpret the financial results.

This note is actually comprised of several smaller parts. The first is the basis of preparation used in the financial statements. This is typically followed by information that supports the numerical data on property and equipment, including depreciation methods. The third part usually discloses the relevant policies and procedures for income tax methods and calculations. These three areas are standard for most medical practices.

However, there may be additional information provided, such as the nature and organization of the business, or other details specific to a particular practice. Our present discussion is limited to the three standard parts: basis of preparation, property and equipment, and income tax.

Basis of Preparation

The first note disclosure usually begins with a description of the basis of financial statement preparation. Since accounting policies and procedures allow for cash basis reporting, accrual basis reporting, or modified cash basis reporting, it is absolutely essential that the financial statements clearly identify which method of accounting and reporting was used.

In Chapter 3, we contrasted the underlying theory, as well as the practical results that occur, when you use the different methods. In Figures 3-6 and 3-7, we showed how the numerical results changed depending on which method of accounting was used. Because correct interpretation of the financial results depends upon understanding the basis of recording, disclosure of this information is normally the first item in this section.

Property and Equipment or Fixed Assets

This part of the note is the most complex because it provides more information than most people can process. Typically, this part of the note can be broken down in a general sense to three smaller components, namely: valuing the asset and the method of depreciation used (including tax depreciation versus financial reporting depreciation); identifying the life of the asset; and policies governing maintenance and repairs.

Because of the complexity and volume of information contained in this note disclosure, we have provided a sample footnote in Figure 6-1, which we will now discuss in detail. This should help you translate the information contained in your own note on property and equipment.

As you can see, there is a tremendous amount of information contained in this sample standard note. Understanding this footnote is extremely important and it

FIGURE 6-1
ILLUSTRATION OF SIGNIFICANT ACCOUNTING POLICIES
GOVERNING DEPRECIATION

Fixed assets are carried at cost. Depreciation is computed for financial reporting purposes using the straight-line method at rates based on estimated useful lives. Depreciation is computed using the rate guidelines established by the Modified Accelerated Cost Recovery System of five and seven years for income tax reporting purposes. In 1993, depreciation was computed using the accelerated system for both financial and income tax purposes. Upon the sale or retirement of assets, the cost and related accumulated depreciation are removed from their respective accounts and the resulting gains or losses included in income. Expenditures for maintenance and repairs are charged to expense as incurred.

combines several of the accounting and reporting concepts discussed throughout the book. If you feel that the terminology is overwhelming, stop periodically and refer to Figure 6-2, a chart which lists the common terms used in this footnote with an easy to understand translation that should keep you focused.

FIGURE 6-2
TERMINOLOGY RELATED TO PROPERTY AND EQUIPMENT

TERMINOLOGY	TRANSLATION
Fixed Assets	Property and equipment
Carried at Cost	Valued at the amount paid to acquire
Estimated Useful Life	How long you expect to use the asset
Straight-Line Method	Spreads the cost of the asset equally over its estimated useful life
Rate Guidelines	Calculation of depreciation by the IRS
Accelerated Depreciation	Higher amounts of depreciation recorded in the earlier years of the asset's life
Modified Accelerated Cost Recovery System (MACRS)	IRS accelerated depreciation method
Financial Reporting Depreciation	Amount of depreciation shown in your financial statements
Income Tax Depreciation	Amount of depreciation shown on your tax return
Maintenance and Repair Expenditures	Amounts necessary for routine upkeep of the asset
Expensed as Incurred	Recorded as an expense when paid

Assets and Their Value

When the note refers to *fixed assets*, they are describing your investment in the property and equipment of the practice. *Fixed assets* is actually an older terminology; the more current term is *property and equipment.*

When the note refers to *carried at cost*, it means that your assets are recorded in the accounting records, and reported in the financial statements, at the original cost you paid to acquire them. This may seem strange since you know that assets are depreciated over time and therefore their value declines. However, the decline in the book value does not affect the original asset account; rather, the decrease in value is reflected in a separate accumulated depreciation account.

Depreciation Methods

Often, two depreciation methods will be used: one for financial reporting purposes and one for income tax preparation. When they refer to financial reporting purposes, they mean the financial statements received from your accountant. When they refer to income tax reporting purposes, they mean the depreciation reported on your tax return filed with the Internal Revenue Service. If the same system was used for both financial reporting and tax purposes, the same number will appear in both places.

The sample note describes depreciation computed for financial reporting purposes using *the straight-line method* at rates based on estimated useful lives. The straight-line method is a generally accepted depreciation method that spreads the cost of the asset equally over its expected useful life. Thus, if you buy equipment that you expect to use for five years (i.e., the estimated useful life), 20 percent of the cost of that asset is converted to expense in each of the next five years.

The footnote also states that depreciation is computed using the rate guidelines established by the Modified Accelerated Cost Recovery System (MACRS) for income tax reporting purposes. These rate guidelines tell you how much tax depreciation can be taken based on the estimated useful life. The guidelines are calculated by the Internal Revenue Service (IRS), using an average for all types of equipment.

When the note refers to MACRS, it means a tax method for calculating depreciation which is allowed by the IRS. This system determines depreciation cost by classifying assets according to a particular type or characteristic.

An *accelerated cost recovery system* simply means that a higher portion of depreciation is recorded in the earlier years of the asset life. This is in contrast to the straight-line method which assumes a constant usage over the life of the asset. Thus, an accelerated cost recovery system recognizes that an asset's value declines more in the earlier years of its use.

The differences between straight-line and accelerated depreciation is easily illustrated with a purchase and subsequent trade-in of a car. Assume you purchased a new car for $25,000 and its estimated useful life is five years. Straight-line depreciation assumes that the value of the car declines $5,000 per year. The accelerated methods assume that the decline in value from year one to year two is actually much greater than the decline from year four to year five. For example, an accelerated method might record

$7,500 as depreciation in year one, while only $2,000 in year five. This situation is certainly well known if you have ever tried to trade in a car after one or two years.

Depreciation Reporting

The sample footnote states that depreciation in 1993 was computed using the accelerated system for both financial and income tax reporting purposes.

Depending on your particular practice, the tax and financial reporting depreciation methods may be the same or they may be different. Because of the different methods, the annual amount of depreciation computed under the accelerated system is not normally the amount of depreciation computed on the straight-line method. In the earlier years of the asset life (i.e., when the asset is newer) the accelerated depreciation amount is higher than the straight-line depreciation. In contrast, the straight-line depreciation amount will be higher than the accelerated method in the last several years of the asset life.

However, you must also recognize that the total dollars depreciated over the life of the asset must be the same, regardless of the method used to calculate depreciation. Thus, the differences between methods are nothing more than a shift in timing between different years as to when the expense is recognized.

Maintenance and Disposal of Assets

Additional information on the sale or retirement of assets, and the expenditures for maintenance and repairs, is also presented in this note. This information is usually easy to understand. If the asset is retired, it must be removed from the accounting records. Likewise, if the asset is sold with a resulting gain or loss on the transaction, the asset is removed from the records and the gain or loss is reported in the current period on the Statement of Revenues and Expenses.

It is also useful to know that maintenance and repairs are charged to expense as incurred. This means that if your practice is on a cash basis of accounting, expenditures for maintenance and repair of property and equipment are expensed whenever payment is made.

The Importance of This Note

The information contained in this note, while complex, is critical because of the differences between tax depreciation methods and depreciation methods used for financial reporting purposes. If a medical practice chooses to depreciate assets on a straight-line basis for financial reporting purposes, but use the faster accelerated methods allowed for tax reporting purposes, it is important that the financial statement reader be aware of these differences in their financial assessment of the practice.

Likewise, the depreciable life of all assets must be considered because there are differences between the depreciable life of one type of asset in contrast to another. For example, depreciation of a fixed asset, such as a building, will occur over a much longer time period than depreciation of medical equipment.

In summary, the chart of terms in Figure 6-2 should help you translate the information contained in this note.

Income Taxes

The last disclosure typically found in the Summary of Significant Accounting Policies is a statement concerning income taxes. This information will vary, depending on your form of organization. For example, a note disclosure for proprietorships and partnerships usually states that the practice is not a separate taxable entity. Therefore, the information flows directly from the medical practice to your personal income tax return.

In contrast, if your medical practice is organized as a corporation, it is a separate taxable entity and additional disclosures are usually shown in a separate footnote on income taxes. This additional disclosure often occurs in cases where there are complexities affecting the income tax status of the corporation.

Debt Disclosures

After the Summary of Significant Accounting Policies, medical practices will usually have a note disclosure that focuses on the debt of the medical practice. This note provides significant supplementary information related to the liabilities reported in the Statement of Assets, Liabilities and Shareholders' Equity.

This footnote tells you whether the amount you owe is short-term debt (i.e., due within one year) or long-term debt (i.e., due after one year). It also tells you to whom the debt is owed, the amount of the required payments, applicable interest rates, and the method used to calculate interest.

The note also identifies any assets that are pledged as collateral for the debt, a schedule of debt by the amount due in each of the next five years, and the amount due in total after those five years. The total interest expense for a particular year might also be noted. This amount should be the same as that reported on the Statement of Revenues and Expenses.

This note disclosure, if appropriate to your practice, actually provides some of the most important information appearing in supplementary form. If you examine the balance sheet, you will typically see only a single amount reported as debt. Yet, the timing of the debt repayment is critical to a medical professional because of cash flow constraints. Thus, knowing not only how much debt is due, but when it is due, is extremely important.

The fact that this footnote disclosure highlights the total interest cost of the debt is also valuable. Without this focus, it is easy to consider interest as just another operating cost. However, when evaluating the true cost of borrowing, this information should always be highlighted.

In summary, if you want to know the total amount of debt due, look at the liability section of the Statement of Assets, Liabilities and Equity. If you want to know when the debt is due, to whom the debt is owed, or what the debt is costing you in terms of interest, you must look at the note disclosure. For purposes of cash flow management, you must always examine the supplemental note disclosure for debt.

Now examine your own note disclosures on debt and see if all of the details mentioned here appear in your own footnote. If they do not, direct your questions to your accountant.

Pension Plan Disclosures

A discussion of pensions could be a book by itself. This is due to both the complexity and importance of this topic. Chapter 9 of this book discusses pensions from a retirement planning perspective. The information presented in this chapter is limited to interpreting the footnote disclosures commonly found in conjunction with your financial statements.

The note disclosure on pension plans attempts to bring together the various elements of the pension puzzle. This is not easy to do since the terminology often confuses people. For a reference guide on terminology, refer to Figure 6-3 throughout this discussion. This chart identifies the commonly used pension terms and provides a corresponding translation for clarification. Understanding the terminology and consideration of the two primary financial components of the pension puzzle in relation to each other, will facilitate your mastery of this footnote.

FIGURE 6-3
PENSION TERMINOLOGY

TERMINOLOGY	TRANSLATION
Accrued pension liability or pension liability	The amount you owe to the pension fund
Pension expense	The cost of the plan for the current time period
Funding policy	How and when payments are made to the pension plan
Defined contribution plan	A pension that specifies the current amount to be deposited with the pension plan
Defined benefit plan	A pension that specifies how much the retiree receives during retirement
Provision for pension expense	Same as pension expense (i.e., the cost of the plan)
Qualified plan	A pension plan that meets IRS regulations
Qualified or eligible employee	Employees who meet the criteria for eligibility established by your pension plan

Financial Components

The first pension component is the *accrued pension liability* shown on the Statement of Assets, Liabilities and Equity. This is the amount of money that the practice owes to the pension plan but has not yet deposited the money with the administrator of the plan.

The second component is the current period *pension expense*. This is the cost of providing a pension plan to the employees in a specific time period. This amount is shown as an expense on the Statement of Revenues and Expenses. Thus, the pension expense is the cost in the current period while the pension liability tells you how much of that cost has not yet been paid.

The amounts reported for the pension liability and pension expense may be the same or they may be different. In cases where the pension liability (what you owe) equals the pension expense (what it cost you), it means that you have not paid the current bill for pensions. Thus, a liability of that amount appears in the current liability section of your Statement of Assets, Liabilities and Equity.

If the pension liability is less than the pension expense, it means that you have not paid all of the current period cost. In contrast, a pension liability in excess of a pension expense, means that the current period expense and some of the prior period costs have not yet been paid.

Whether or not a liability exists depends on the practice's policy with respect to *funding* the pension plan. Funding describes the process by which the assets needed to pay the retirees are accumulated in the pension plan. This is the same process involved in saving for your child's college education. You must first estimate the amount needed for their tuition payments. You then determine the amount you must deposit today and in the upcoming years to accumulate (including interest earned on the fund) the total needed when they reach college age.

Pension plan funding works the same way. The typical funding sources are periodic cash deposits and interest that is earned and accumulates. If your pension plan requires full annual funding of the expense, there should be no pension liability since the deposits to the pension fund have been made.

In cases where the pension liability is more than the pension expense, not only was the current period pension expense not paid, a portion of the pension expense from a prior year also was not paid. This situation does not normally occur in a medical practice.

Pension Plan Options

The note disclosure on pensions also provides information on the various options that a pension plan may contain. These options are: the type of pension plan, the employees covered by that plan, and a statement of the plan's funding policy.

Medical practices that provide a pension plan normally use a defined contribution plan. In this type of plan, the medical practice makes a specified and fixed amount of contribution to the plan as part of the employee benefits package. This type of plan is the opposite of a defined benefit plan, where the amount of benefits paid at retirement is fixed.

When your footnote disclosure makes reference to a plan covering all "eligible" or "qualified" employees, it means that any of your employees who meet certain specified criteria, as defined in the plan document, are covered by the plan. Qualified or eligible employees are judged against the specifics of your particular pension plan, which in turn had to meet certain criteria defined by the IRS in order to be classified as "qualified." The relevant criteria focus on length of service, full-time or part-time status, and other equity criteria.

The selection of a funding option by the practice is the third disclosure in the pension plan footnote. As we mentioned earlier, funding is the actual deposit of cash with the pension plan. Another way to view funding is the segregation of assets which will be used to pay benefits after the employee retires.

This note disclosure often states that the plan will be funded via contributions based on employee compensation. It may also state that all pension expense for a given time period will be funded. In this case, the practice deposits an amount equal to the pension cost for the period. Therefore, no corresponding liability will appear on the Statement of Assets, Liabilities and Equity because the deposits have been made to the pension fund.

Understanding Pension Disclosures

The footnote on pensions is needed because it gives you valuable operating information that cannot be reduced to a number in the financial statements. For example, the funding policy is important because it requires an annual commitment of cash. There is questionable benefit to a pension plan if you do not deposit the cash necessary to ensure that assets are available to pay the needed pension benefits when employees retire. Thus, to assess a medical practice's ability and willingness to meet the pension obligations, clear statements on funding provisions must be made.

Another commonly used term in the pension footnote is the phrase *provision for pension expense*. This is another way of saying the pension expense or current period costs for the plan. This terminology is also commonly used in the area of income taxes, which will be discussed shortly.

It is also beneficial to have the note disclosure clearly identify the total pension expense for the period. Depending on your financial statement, pension expense may be shown in more than one place. For example, a medical practice may separately categorize their costs for partners, and their costs for other employees of the practice. In this situation, pension expense for each of these two components will appear in two different places in the Statement of Revenue and Expense. Thus, to assess the total impact of pension costs on the financial situation of the practice, you should always refer to the footnote disclosure on pensions.

A summary of the common pension terms appears in Figure 6-3 for your reference.

Leases and Related Party Transactions

Leasing can be an important issue. For example, assume that you are considering the purchase of an existing medical practice. One of the reasons you are interested in this particular practice is because of their lower monthly operating expenses compared to another practice that is for sale. As part of your analysis, you ask for the financial statements, including note disclosures.

When you receive the information, you analyze their Statement of Revenues and Expenses and verify that their rent expense for their office is indeed quite low, relative to what you are currently paying. You think it would be a great deal if you were able to continue their rental agreement. You are just about ready to pursue this purchase option when your associate asks for information on the owner of the medical building from which that practice leases their facilities.

You tell him that such information is not available in the financial statements. He acknowledges that fact and he suggests that you read the footnote disclosures on leases and related party transactions. In doing so, you discover that the medical practice that is for sale is the majority shareholder in a real estate venture that owns the medical building and that the lease rates are only good between the existing parties. In other words, you now have good reason to believe that if you buy the practice, the existing rates will not apply to you.

This information could have easily been overlooked if your associate didn't recognize the significance of leases and related party transactions. Disclosure of lease information is common because many medical practices rent their office facilities. Disclosure of related party transactions is required so that the financial statement reader is aware of the personal and/or financial relationships that exist between and among individuals or groups with a vested interest in the medical practice.

For businesses other than medical practices, lease and related party information appears as two separate footnotes. However, this information is often presented together for medical practices because the rental often occurs in conjunction with another organization in which a physician or several physicians have a vested ownership interest.

It is important to know about these relationships because leases are a commitment of future cash flows by the medical practice. It is also important to disclose when individual partners have a vested interest in the success of a financial venture that is directly related to the operation of the medical practice.

This footnote has become more important in recent years because many practices now have satellite or second operating offices. These additional offices are a result of the need for geographical outreach to better serve patients or as an attempt to attract new patients in an increasingly competitive marketplace.

The significance of this note has also increased because many physicians have invested in financial ventures, some of which are real estate partnerships. These financial arrangements often are investments in buildings or other medical facilities that the physicians' patients may or may not use.

This note typically tells you the "minimum future lease payments." You need to know this amount because the medical practice has committed to these payments in the future to satisfy the lease obligation. Yet, this commitment is not recorded as a liability in the financial records. This situation is often referred to as "off–balance sheet financing" because the liability exists but is not reported in the financial statements. Thus, the minimum future lease payments indicate the maximum financial exposure that the practice has in the event that there is an attempt to end the lease.

Disclosure of lease information becomes more valuable if the medical practice has more than one lease arrangement. In this case, the note disclosure normally identifies (1) the individual leases, (2) the facilities to which the lease relates, and (3) the amount of the monthly financing commitment. In addition, this note tells you whether any individual partner, or partners in the medical group, have a direct ownership interest.

When lease obligations are related to a vested financial interest by any member of the medical practice, this note is of increased interest. Of prime importance is whether or not the payments made by the medical practice are at a fair market value (i.e., what the owner of the facility would charge to any unrelated party using the property). This is an area of particular interest to the IRS who seeks proof that rental payments between related parties are at fair market value.

Income Taxes

As we mentioned earlier, a medical practice organized as a proprietorship or a partnership is not a separate taxable entity. Disclosing the tax status for proprietorships and partnerships is normally part of the first capstone note, the disclosure of significant accounting policies.

However, if the medical practice is organized as a corporation, it is a separate taxable entity and income taxes are shown in the financial statements of the medical practice. With a corporate form of organization, the tax status of the medical practice becomes more complicated and the note disclosure on income taxes is an attempt to clarify the tax situation.

Financial Statement Tax Elements

This note disclosure typically refers to a *provision for income taxes*. This is simply another way of saying the current period expense and is comparable to the provision for pensions discussed earlier. The provision for income taxes is shown on the Statement of Revenues and Expenses.

The footnote also discloses the amount of taxes due to the IRS that have not yet been paid. This liability is typically seen in the current liabilities section of the Statement of Assets, Liabilities and Equity. If none of the provision for income taxes has been paid, the amount of income tax expense on the Statement of Revenues and Expenses will equal the tax liability on the Statement of Assets, Liabilities and Equity. However, since most corporations make quarterly estimated tax payments, you will not usually see a tax liability that equals the provision for income taxes.

Carry-Forward Provisions

The income tax note disclosure also tells you whether there are any tax *carry-forwards*. Carry-forwards occur when the corporation is unable to use all of the tax benefits allowed under the tax law in a given year. Carry-forwards are a benefit that can be used in future years with certain specified limits. The most common carry-forward provisions affecting corporate medical practices are: net operating loss carry-forwards, Section 179 carry-forwards, and contribution carry-forwards.

Operating loss carry-forwards occur because corporations do not get a tax refund if they have a loss for the period; yet they owe taxes if they generate income. The carry-forward provision allows them to use the loss from one year to offset the income in subsequent years. To illustrate, assume that a medical practice loses $50,000 in its first year of operations. The corporation would have a zero tax bill in this year but would not receive a tax refund. In year two, assume the practice has $200,000 of income. The carry-forward provision allows them to take the $50,000 loss from year one and offset it against the $200,000 income from year two. Thus, their taxable income in year two would be $150,000 even though the actual reported income is $200,000.

In our example above, we assumed that the loss occurred in year one of the business. In contrast, let's assume a loss in year 10. The tax laws for operating losses actually have two pieces, a carry-back and a carry-forward provision.

Therefore, if the loss occurred in year 10, you would recalculate the prior three years' tax liability, using the loss as a reduction of the income in those years. Any unused amount can then be carried forward in the same way as the example noted above. Businesses do have the option to forego the carry-back provision and only use the carry-forward option. This is done when there is a better tax benefit to be obtained in future years.

A Section 179 carry-forward arises when the practice was unable to take maximum advantage of Section 179 of the IRS code. This section allows businesses to write off as expense, purchases of equipment in an amount up to $17,500 (under current regulations). Expensing the equipment rather than capitalizing it and reflecting it on the balance sheet where it is depreciated over several years, means faster tax benefits are realized. Thus, using Section 179 expense provides an immediate tax benefit to the practice. If a medical practice is unable to use all of this benefit in a particular year due to other regulations related to Section 179 (see Chapter 5), the unused portion may be carried forward to offset taxes in subsequent years.

A contribution carry-forward arises when the corporation actually makes charitable contributions in excess of the amount allowed under IRS regulations. These excess contributions can be carried forward and classified as a contribution in a subsequent year.

Regardless of the type of carry-forward, the expiration date of the benefits, as well as the amount of the benefit, will be disclosed in the footnote. Since tax carry-forwards are typically available to offset future tax liabilities, the note disclosure will tell you how they will be reflected in the financial statements at the point when they are actually used.

Accounts Receivable

In an earlier discussion, we described how cash or modified cash basis accounting records revenues only when cash is received. If you provide services for patients but are not paid at the time of service, a receivable exists for the practice. However, under cash or modified cash basis reporting, the receivable is not reflected in the financial statements.

For medical practices that use cash basis reporting, the note on accounts receivable will typically disclose the amount due to the practice from patients or third party insurers. This information is usually reported because the amount is not shown in the financial statement, but it represents future cash inflows to the medical practice.

However, if your medical practice uses the accrual basis of accounting, accounts receivable is reported in the current assets section of the Statement of Assets, Liabilities and Equity. The receivables are reported in the amount that has been billed to patients, whether they will be paid by the patient or a third party insurer.

Under the accrual method of accounting, you must also estimate any accounts receivable that you think you will be unable to collect. This estimate is known as the *allowance for bad debts* and it reduces the value of accounts receivable. If you are under the accrual method of accounting, the note disclosure typically defines which method was used to estimate bad debts, as well as the amount of bad debt expense recognized in a given time period.

The note disclosures described in the previous pages are those that are common to most medical practices. However, there may be additional disclosures particular to your individual practice. If you have a question on any of the note disclosures in your own financial report, it would be wise to direct those questions to your accountant at your next meeting.

The information found in typical note disclosures has been summarized in Figure 6-4. This should serve as a quick reference for you to determine how and where specific information is reported.

How Footnote Information Is Useful in Managing Your Medical Practice

A note disclosure meets the objective of good financial reporting because it gathers information that appears in various places in the financial statements, shows the interrelationships, summarizes the information, and presents it as one related and comprehensive set of facts. Therefore, it allows you to see how the pieces of a particular puzzle fit together. Use these note disclosures as an opportunity to master the more difficult financial aspects of your practice.

FIGURE 6-4
SUMMARY OF INFORMATION CONTAINED IN THE NOTE DISCLOSURES

FOOTNOTE	INFORMATION
Summary of Significant Accounting Policies	Basis of accounting used Depreciable lives of property Depreciation methods used Form of organization Maintenance and repair policy Sale/disposals of property Taxability status
Debt or Notes Payable	Amount of debt, short-term Amount of debt, long-term Collateral pledged Debtor Interest expense Interest rate Payments required Timing of debt payments
Pension Plan	Contributions to Employees covered Funding of pension Pension expense Pension liability Provision for pension Type of pension plan
Lease Commitments/Related Party Transactions	Minimum future lease payments—total Monthly lease amount Ownership percentage in related party arrangements Related parties
Income Taxes	Financial statement treatment Income tax expense Income tax payable Loss carry-forwards—amount Loss carry-forwards—type Prepaid taxes Tax liability Provision for taxes
Accounts Receivable	*Accounting method used for bad debts *Allowance for bad debts Amount due from patients and insurance companies

* Accrual basis only

Good management of a medical practice also requires a view toward the "big picture." Focusing on the financial statements alone leaves a gap in the information necessary for good decision making. Including the note disclosures in your analysis of your financial results gives you the complete picture.

The type of information that appears in the note disclosures is critical but cannot always be reduced to a number that appears in financial statements. The notes also show information that is a numerical result but is not reported in the financial statements because of other factors. Evaluation of this information will help you to determine if all of the pieces of the puzzle are considered in your decision-making process. This focus should also allow you to determine whether there is a consistency among and between the financial elements in the practice.

Thus, to have complete information for good business decisions, you must analyze the note disclosures in conjunction with the financial statement results.

Physician's Checklist

As a summary of this chapter, ask yourself the following questions with respect to note disclosures. If you can answer "yes" to these questions, you have a good understanding of financial statement disclosures.

_____ 1. Do you know how often you receive footnote disclosures in conjunction with your financial statements?

_____ 2. Does your accountant review this information with you?

_____ 3. Do you know which note disclosures are presented?

_____ 4. Do you understand the information contained in the individual notes?

_____ 5. Do you use this information as an aid in analyzing your financial results?

_____ 6. Do you know what your significant accounting policies are and how they impact financial accounting and reporting in your medical practice?

_____ 7. Can you identify your debt repayment schedules with respect to the amount and when it is due?

_____ 8. Can you identify any additional information that you need that does not appear in either the financial statements or the accompanying note disclosures?

If you answered "yes" to these questions, you should be comfortable with the financial affairs of your business. You can now proceed to Chapter 7, which discusses a critical operating component of your business, protecting your business assets.

Questions and Answers

1. **What should I do with the narrative information that accompanies the annual financial report received from my accountant?**

    The narrative information received with your annual report gives you additional explanations for the numerical results reported in your financial statement. In addition, they describe and provide information about other aspects of your financial policies, such as how your accounting policies impact the reporting of financial events, how your pension plan is funded, etc. Attention should be paid to this information.

7 Protecting Your Business Assets

Dr. Lave faces a dilemma. His long-time bookkeeper left the practice several weeks ago when her husband accepted a new job and they relocated in another state. When the new bookkeeper began work, Dr. Lave suggested that she review the past several months of accounting records as a way to familiarize herself with her job responsibilities.

After several days, the new bookkeeper hesitantly approaches Dr. Lave with a problem. She thinks that the old bookkeeper may have prepared refund checks for nonexistent patients and cashed the checks herself. Dr. Lave states that it's impossible because the checks were always signed by him and he always examined the patient accounts receivable ledger card attached to the refund request. The new bookkeeper explains that she recognized one of the patient's names but didn't think that she was a patient of Dr. Lave. Although it was inappropriate, she decided to look for her friend's medical file. When she couldn't find it in the active drawer, she looked in the inactive files. However, no file existed.

The new bookkeeper also noticed similar handwriting on the endorsements of another refund check and decided to see if that patient file existed. Once again she looked in both the active and inactive files but couldn't locate a medical file. The new bookkeeper then checked all patient refund checks for that month and discovered that three of the 10 checks had endorsements with similar handwriting and no medical file.

After he got over his initial shock and confusion, Dr. Lave thought about his involvement in the process and realized that in many cases, he simply signed the checks in between seeing patients and gave only cursory attention to the task. He didn't think anything of it at the time, but he realizes now that his patient base is quite large and a photocopy of a simple ledger card with numbers on it didn't mean anything as supporting documentation. He should have asked for more. . . .

Dr. Lave thinks about his current problem and realizes that as his practice grew, he delegated more and more responsibility to the bookkeeper and never thought about the need to monitor or control what she did. Now he realizes that he must learn how to protect his cash and other business assets, as well as devising controls over how the accounting records are processed. He decides to call his accountant to schedule a meeting regarding the policies and procedures he might use to protect himself and the assets of the business.

To help Dr. Lave in his quest for knowledge on internal controls, this chapter will answer several questions:

- What are internal controls?
- Why are internal controls often ignored by medical practitioners?
- What constitutes good internal control?
- Why are they important to a medical practice?
- What role does a physician play in the control structure?
- What specific controls can be used to protect business assets?
- How can internal controls be implemented if there are only a few employees?
- What level of internal control is present in your medical practice?

What Are Internal Controls?

Internal controls are the policies and procedures which ensure that your business assets are used properly and accounted for correctly. Policies are the general guidelines that govern your operating environment; procedures are the specific tasks you use to accomplish a particular control objective effectively. For example, an internal control policy requires that you separate the individual who writes checks from the individual who enters the transactions in the records. In contrast, an internal control procedure requires that you stamp "paid" on the bills supporting a request for payment.

Physicians typically have no background in internal controls and in some cases, lack direct knowledge of the policies and procedures used in their own office. Later in this chapter, we will detail the specific procedures you can use to protect your business assets. However, if you remember the three general policies noted below, you can apply them to any aspect of your operating and financial environment. These three general policies are: (1) segregate job responsibilities, (2) require authorizations and approvals of transactions, and (3) periodically reconcile information.

Segregating job responsibilities means separating the individual who has access to any form of assets (e.g., cash including checks) from the individual who processes the paperwork. Not only will this prevent a person from removing the asset and altering the supporting record, it also assigns specific responsibility for the transaction.

The second general policy requires that you implement an authorization and approval process. This policy usually requires two steps; the first is that you designate specific events or transactions which need authorization, and the second is that you identify the physician responsible for a particular area. This requires that you take an active role in the approval process; don't simply sign any document presented to you. We recognize that this is a real constraint on physicians' time. However, we recommend that you establish a routine procedure for processing documents, which includes how and when they are presented to you for approval. This will ensure that nothing unintended gets your signature.

The third internal control policy is periodic reconciliation. This means that on a **routine** and **regular** interval, a designated individual examines the records that support the financial transactions. For example, you should review the detailed accounts receivable list, and determine that it agrees with the total accounts receivable reported, on a monthly basis.

Although these general internal controls appear to be common sense, they are often overlooked. However, they can be effectively implemented with minimal effort in your medical practice. Later in the chapter, we will detail specific internal control procedures and show you how they relate to your medical practice's accounting and administrative functions.

Why Are Internal Controls Often Ignored?

The development and use of internal controls have not received the attention they deserve, particularly in small medical practices. This is not unusual because most physicians believe that they do not have enough employees to consider the use of internal controls. We recognize that the smaller the number of employees, the more difficult it is to implement internal controls. However, there are certain controls that can be used effectively, even in small practices.

The costs associated with the design, implementation, and maintenance of internal controls is another reason why they are often ignored by medical practices. While physicians understand the costs associated with controls, it is often difficult to clearly identify and measure the benefits they provide, until it is too late. Typically, the benefits of internal controls are only understood after a crisis has arisen that highlights the need for, or the abuse of, internal control practices.

The third reason medical practices don't consider internal controls to be a pressing concern is the competing time demands physicians face in managing the medical practice. The issue of internal controls is normally at the bottom of the priority list of operating issues for physicians. This is particularly true in smaller medical practices that do not employ an office manager. Although these concerns are understandable, you must consider internal control an issue worthy of your time.

Medical practices with a stable work force are particularly susceptible to ignoring internal controls. This is true because the more stable the work force, the more comfortable everyone is with the daily operating activities. This comfort level can often take the form of a family atmosphere in the medical practice, and as a result, a great deal of trust is placed in the employees. However, a significant number of embezzle-ments have been perpetrated by the "trusted" employee.

As medical practices continue to evolve into businesses, they need to be managed as such, and internal controls must be a top priority.

Why Are Internal Controls Important?

Despite the constraints noted above, internal controls are critical for your business. Remember that when we discuss internal controls, we are talking about controls over both the record-keeping process and over the asset itself. Without controls, you cannot be sure that your financial transactions are processed correctly, or in accordance with your authorization and intent. Without such assurance, the data produced by your information system may not be reliable. If the data are not reliable, you cannot make good business decisions.

Internal controls are also important in managing and safeguarding the assets of your practice. Without proper control over your resources, there is nothing to prevent your employees from using your business assets to their personal benefit. Taking this idea further, you must realize that without some form of internal control, there is little to protect you from an employee who wants to take an asset from your business.

The ability of your medical practice to successfully develop and implement internal controls is governed by your attitude toward the importance of these controls. Therefore, you must create an environment that promotes the development, implementation, maintenance, and support of policies and procedures that provide this safety mechanism.

In the following pages, you will see a large number of relatively simple things that can be done to improve control over both your record-keeping process and your assets. Many of these controls do not require substantial reorganization of your office, nor cause significant additional costs. Although many of these policies and procedures are simple, in most cases, they will be effective in preventing problems.

A word of caution is appropriate at this time. Although a properly designed system of internal accounting controls can go a long way in protecting your business, it is not a 100 percent guarantee. This is particularly true in a small practice with a limited number of employees. However, time and costs incurred are well worth the effort if they prevent the possible misuse of your business assets.

Your Role in Internal Control

If you remember nothing else from this chapter, remember your role in the development and management of internal control procedures. **Never forget that the *best* internal control is *your* keen oversight of the financial and operating transactions in your practice.**

We recognize that this is a difficult task for a physician, particularly one who is a sole practitioner or one who manages a large medical practice. However, it is critical that you use your oversight role daily. Many recent cases involving small business fraud have shown that it could have been minimized, if not prevented, had the individual responsible for oversight been actively involved in the events of the business. Although there are competing demands for your time, and you may delegate the more routine office functions to others, you must make a conscious effort to actively participate and supervise the financial affairs of your business.

Standard Control Procedures

Internal control policies are general in nature and are used to shape the operating environment in your business. Internal control procedures are specific tasks you can use to provide some form of asset protection.

However, you must also realize that no single control procedure will prevent all problems. Rather, you usually need a combination of several controls to be effective. For example, if you don't have a control that requires the individual who processes the cash to be different from the employee who records the accounting information, the effectiveness of many of the other procedures is limited.

In addition, you must note that some of the internal control procedures are preventative in nature, some are detection oriented, while others have both capabilities. To illustrate, requiring two signatures on checks over a certain dollar value is designed to prevent large transactions from being processed unless it is authorized and reviewed by two people.

In contrast, accounting for the numbering sequence is detection oriented since it would identify unauthorized use of a document. Meanwhile, requiring that invoices be canceled by stamping "paid" across the bill prevents it from being processed for payment a second time and it is easy to detect such an attempt because you have defaced the bill.

Many of the procedures described in the next section are easy to put in place and do not require significant additional costs to your business.

Use Only Prenumbered Documents

Using only prenumbered documents for any transaction in the practice is a standard internal control procedure. *Documents* include obvious things, such as patients' receipts or checks, but should also be used for purchase orders and receiving documents.

Prenumbered documents let you to trace and verify any transaction within your system. However, you can also identify unauthorized use of documents if you see gaps in the numbering sequence. To detect this, you must periodically verify the numerical sequence. Although use of prenumbered documents is usually standard procedure, part of its control value is destroyed if you don't account for the numerical sequence at periodic intervals.

To ensure proper accounting for sequential documents, you must keep all voided copies. Further control over documents requires that they be issued only to those who have proper authority and that you restrict access to any unused forms.

Cancel Documents

A simple, yet effective, control procedure in the area of cash disbursements is the cancellation of supporting documentation when a bill is paid. Physicians routinely sign checks and return the supporting invoices and checks to the office manager who prepared them. Supporting documents should not be returned unless the invoices have been marked paid, with the appropriate check number noted on the bill.

Canceling the document accomplishes two things. First, it leaves a trail by which the payment can be verified if questions arise. Second, it makes it easy to detect if the same invoice is submitted for payment twice. Thus, when you examine the supporting documentation for cash payments, simply stamp "paid" on the face of the invoice to prevent further reprocessing.

Compare Documents

Comparing documents is a simple and effective control procedure and should be done while you are signing the checks. You can do this by comparing the original bill or invoice to the actual check for both the amount of the check and the individual or company to whom the check is written.

You should also compare the information on the bill to the information on the purchase order and receiving document, verifying the quantity, type of merchandise, invoice amount, and payment terms. This comparison prevents you from paying for the wrong type of merchandise, an incorrect quantity of merchandise, or the wrong amount. It also insures payment consistent with the agreed-upon terms. Using these controls means you should never pay for merchandise you didn't receive.

Any discrepancies noted between the supporting documentation and the check, or between the invoice and other supporting documents, should immediately be investigated. This requires particular attention if the discrepancies are with the check payee, the quantity of merchandise, or the amount of the check.

Process Information on a Forward-Only Basis

A simple rule to remember when dealing with internal control and document processing is: records or documentation should flow forward, not backward. By this we mean that once an individual has prepared or had access to a transaction, and it is passed through to the next level for authorization or signature, don't return it to the original preparer.

A good example of this control is the check signing function within cash disbursements. Once you compare the documents and stamp them "paid," sign the checks but don't return them to the individual who prepared them. Rather, give the checks to the receptionist for mailing and give the supporting canceled documents to another individual for filing. By not returning the checks and supporting documentation to the individuals who prepared them, you prevent their alteration after they have your approval and signature.

Use Double Signatures

Requiring two signatures on checks is a very effective internal control procedure. Although this is not possible for solo practitioners and is difficult for small group practices, you should consider whether this control could be implemented effectively into your practice. The larger the medical practice, the more benefit this control provides.

You don't need to require double signatures on all checks. Rather, checks over a certain dollar value, whose amount needs to be determined by your individual practice, should require duplicate signatures. With this control, checks cannot be cashed by the payee without two signatures, which means that at least two individuals reviewed the documentation and approved the payment. Whether the dual signatures should be two physicians, or an office manager and one physician, is a decision that has to be made by your practice. However, this control is excellent in providing additional security over major cash disbursements.

Require Documentation for All Purchases

All purchases made by the medical practice should be validated with some form of documentation. Using *purchase orders* easily accomplishes this. A purchase order is a prenumbered document that indicates the same information on the supplier's bill or invoice (i.e., vendor name and address, quantity and type of merchandise ordered, dollar amount of the purchase, and the agreed-upon payment terms). A copy of the purchase order (without the quantity ordered noted, to force the individual receiving the merchandise to actually count it) can then be used as a receiving document. Using a receiving document substantiates the actual receipt of goods by your practice.

While purchase orders protect your practice by documenting the type and quantity that you ordered, at the agreed-upon terms, a receiving document verifies the receipt of the actual goods. Although this may seem unnecessary for small purchases, such as supplies, there is only a minimal cost to using purchase orders and receiving documents for all acquisitions. In safeguarding your assets, the benefits obtained certainly outweigh the minimal cost incurred. You should also require advance authorization and approval of purchase orders over a certain dollar value.

Obtain Bids for Purchases of Equipment

As noted above, the use of purchase orders and receiving documents substantiate and validate your purchases. Using these documents is particularly important for the more significant purchases, such as office or medical equipment.

When acquiring office or medical equipment, it is a good policy to require written bids, with pricing, for such purchases. This helps to ensure that the proper and best purchasing decision was made. The purchase should then be substantiated by the use of a purchase order, receiving document, etc., noted earlier.

Separate Jobs to Assign Responsibility

The receipt of cash is one area where internal controls are critical. Therefore, you should use all available procedures to provide maximum protection over cash. The first control you can implement is to separate cash when it is received from its supporting documentation. This means that the receptionist who accepts payment from the patient, or opens the mail and receives checks from the insurance company, should immediately separate the cash from its supporting documentation (e.g., the remittance advice or a copy of the statement). The receptionist can then process the cash for deposit.

Meanwhile, the documentation received in support of the cash received, should be processed by a second individual for entry into the accounting system. Thus, you have separated the cash from its supporting documentation and used two individuals, each responsible for a particular part of the process. The total of the receipts processed by each individual can then be compared by you or another individual designated by you. This will insure that the amount processed is correct.

Separating the processing of cash from its supporting documentation prevents an employee from removing both the cash and its paperwork. If they are able to remove both the asset and its supporting documentation, it is almost impossible to detect the theft. However, with the separation of jobs, any attempt to remove cash will be detected when the amount of cash receipts reported by the first employee does not agree with the amount of cash receipts determined by the second individual.

Process Transactions on a Timely Basis

Good internal control requires timely processing of financial transactions. This is particularly true in the area of cash and it means that you should deposit cash daily. While cash is in the office, access to it must be restricted. To minimize potential problems in this area, cash should be removed from the office and deposited in the bank daily.

Although timely processing seems obvious, there are businesses that allow cash to remain in the office for several days, without being processed or deposited. You should not delay processing transactions or depositing cash because an employee is out sick or on vacation. There should always be a second individual who can perform another's job responsibilities.

Restrict Access

Restricting access to both the asset and its supporting documentation is a requirement of good internal control. Applying this means using a locked drawer or safe for cash, limiting those with access to office or medical supplies, using passwords for computer entry, and limiting the number of individuals who can enter data into the accounting records.

Restricting access also includes minimizing the number of people who have keys to the cash box. In addition, other assets and the accounting records should be physically restricted in an area that can effectively be closed off to those who do not have authority within that function.

Reconcile Assets to Their Supporting Records

For asset protection, you must periodically verify the existence of your assets. You must also determine that the accounting records agree with the assets that you know exist. This should be done monthly for accounts receivable and cash, and at least annually for office supplies inventory, medical supplies inventory, and equipment of the medical practice.

Good cash control requires that bank reconcilements for all cash accounts be performed monthly, by individuals other than those who have access to cash. This means that any employee who makes deposits, writes checks, or has signature authority should not perform the reconcilement function.

The reconcilement process is also important for medical and office supplies, particularly if no record-keeping is used when supplies are taken from the storeroom. Only through periodic counting of inventory, in connection with restricted access to the inventory, will you maintain good control over supplies.

Reconciling the medical and office equipment to the supporting accounting records should also be performed to determine that the assets are properly accounted for. This can be done annually by using serial numbers on computers, printers, typewriters, and medical equipment.

Actively Manage Accounts Receivable

Without internal controls, proper management of accounts receivable is difficult. This is particularly true for patient refunds or write-offs of uncollectible accounts. These matters require close oversight by the physician since it is an area that is relatively easy to manipulate. Specifically, your active management and attention to supporting details makes it easier to detect if an employee pockets a payment from a patient and then writes-off or deletes the account receivable.

The easiest control over refunds and write-offs is the requirement authorization from a designated physician. However, this necessitates your willingness to take an active role in managing this process. Therefore, you must review the records and supporting documentation to determine that an account is actually uncollectible or that the patient is due to receive a refund. Additional policies and procedures must also be used to prevent the theft of funds from an account that you wrote off as uncollectible, but subsequently received the cash from a patient.

Bond Employees Who Handle Cash

A standard internal control is to *bond* all employees who handle cash. Bonding is the purchase of an insurance policy to protect you against employee theft. As part of the process, the bonding companies usually perform background checks on the employees prior to bonding them.

Thus, bonding is a good control because it acts as a deterrent to theft and it also is good business sense because it is an insurance policy in the event theft occurs. Bonding employees who handle cash is a standard practice in any business.

Summary of Controls

In each of the areas discussed above, we tried to show how simple, but effective, control mechanisms are used to manage and protect your medical practice assets. Most of these procedures can be implemented with little additional cost to the practice. What these procedures do require is a little bit of thought and your willingness to recognize their importance in protecting your assets.

As a summary, Figure 7-1 includes the internal control procedures discussed in this chapter, as well as a brief description of what each control accomplishes. We recommend that you read the list and check off the procedures you presently use in your practice. Then focus on those that you don't use and determine the best way they can be implemented.

Get Involved!

We recognize that your practice may be too small even for some of the basic controls noted above. If this is the case, remember the following rule: the smaller the practice, the fewer internal controls you have and therefore, the greater your role in internal control. This means that you must actively perform an oversight role, particularly in the area of cash receipts and disbursements. It is not enough to rely on your accountant! Remember the role and responsibility of your accountant described in Chapter 1? If you have compilation services performed, their task is normally limited to processing your

---

FIGURE 7-1
INTERNAL CONTROL SUMMARY

Internal Control Procedure	What Problem Does It Prevent or Detect?
Use only prenumbered documents	Invalid transactions
Account for numerical sequence	Unauthorized use
Cancel documents	Paying a bill twice
Compare documents	Payment for the wrong merchandise
Use forward-only processing	Altering documents after their initial processing
Use double signatures for large expenditures	Sole authority for large or significant expenditures
Require documentation of purchases	Invalid transactions
Obtain written bids for equipment or other major purchases	Incorrect purchasing decision
Separate job functions	Asset removal and subsequent cover-up using the related accounting records
Timely processing	Inaccurate record-keeping
Restrict access to assets and financial records	Use by unauthorized individuals
Reconcile assets to records	Nonagreement between the physical asset and its supporting accounting record
Require physician approval for patient refunds and write-offs	Invalid transactions
Bond employees who handle cash	Employee theft of cash

---

financial information in financial statement format. It does not include a review or assessment of your operating policies and procedures.

We know that it is difficult to discuss internal controls as a preventative measure since everyone thinks that their employees are honest. In fact, that is how problems occur. The potential for employee fraud requires your attention, particularly since reports of white collar crime have increased in recent years. Internal controls serve a second purpose because they help assure an accurate processing of your information. Without accurate processing, the resulting output is flawed and incorrect business decisions can result.

The internal control procedures noted above are not usually used individually. In fact, many of them are combined and applied to the various accounting areas. To illustrate, we will now examine your cash receipts and cash disbursements functions (a substantial majority of your daily accounting activity), and show you how the individual controls are combined and implemented within those functions. We will begin with a flowchart illustrating the transaction and document flow within each area (see Figures 7-2 and 7-3). We will then highlight where controls can be placed and which controls work in tandem in these operating areas (see Figures 7-4 and 7-5).

We recognize that many medical practices are small and that the number of employees may not be conducive to the design and implementation of control procedures. However, note that only three individuals were needed to function effectively and provide a degree of control over the assets of the practice.

Internal Controls over the Cash Receipt Function

The cash receipts cycle for any business begins with the receipt of cash or a check. In your medical practice, the cycle begins either with payment by a patient in the office or with the receipt of checks from insurance companies or patients in the daily mail. Either way the process is basically the same.

It is also important to note that when we talk about cash receipts, we are talking about cash or checks. Although there is a tendency to think of checks as more secure than cash, let us caution you that many frauds in the work environment have involved checks. The need to alter checks is not a particularly significant deterrent to anyone trying to steal your money.

For maximum control over cash receipts, it is important that the document which supports the cash received be separated from the actual cash or check as soon as possible. For receipt of checks through the mail, one employee should open and sort the contents into two piles immediately. The first pile should contain the checks that have been received; the second should contain either the remittance advice or a copy of the bill or statement paid by the patient or insurance company.

The checks should be totaled and processed for deposit immediately. This means stamping "for deposit only" on the back of the check. This restrictive endorsement indicates that the checks should only be deposited in the account noted, not cashed for any individual. Meanwhile, the remittance advices should be totaled simultaneously and used for data entry into the accounting records.

FIGURE 7-2
CASH RECEIPTS CYCLE TRANSACTION AND DOCUMENT FLOW

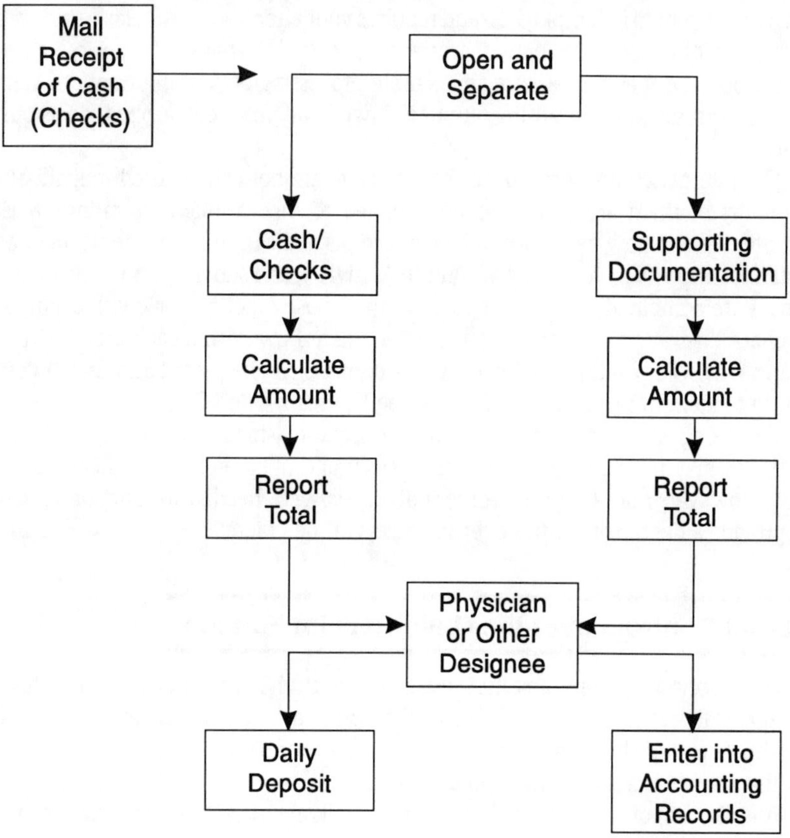

The individual processing the cash and the individual processing the remittance advices, should separately report the total value of their records to a third individual. This provides a check at the point of receipt and verifies that the cash for deposit and the supporting records are equal in amount at that point in time.

Once the cash is totaled and the amount agrees with the supporting documentation, a deposit slip should be prepared accordingly. The deposit should be taken to the bank before the end of the day.

Cash or checks received from patients in the office can be handled the same way. However, implicit in the office set-up is a secondary control over cash receipts (i.e., the patient). This control takes place when the receptionist gives a copy of the doctor's bill to the patient.

FIGURE 7-3
CASH DISBURSEMENTS TRANSACTION AND DOCUMENT FLOW

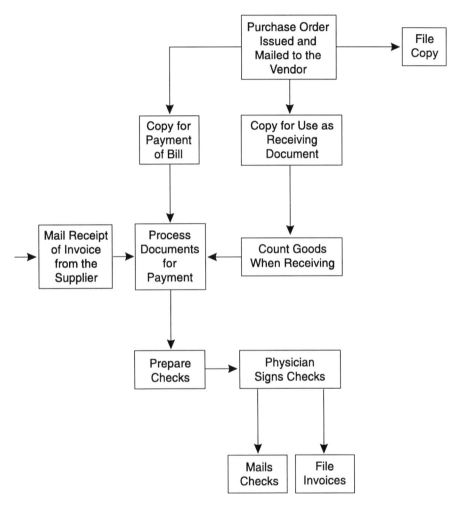

Further control over the cash receipts function (and simultaneously the cash disbursement function) requires that a monthly bank reconcilement be performed by an individual who has not had any direct access to the cash or the supporting accounting records.

Let's take a minute now and consider which internal controls were used in our description of the cash receipts cycle. First, a receipt should be used to document all services rendered and the receipt should be prenumbered. Second, we illustrated separation of duties when we described separating the cash from the supporting documents at the point of receipt. Separation of duties is also used when a third individual prepares the monthly bank reconcilement. Thus, the reconcilement process was also used.

We also used comparison of information when we asked that the cash amounts be reported separately by the individual preparing cash, and the individual processing the accounting records. Last but not least, we required timely deposit of cash and record processing.

In addition, we discussed the value of using prenumbered documents and accounting for the numbering sequence. Accounting for the prenumbered documents is a valuable internal control. To illustrate, consider the following example.

A patient is seen in the office and stops at the receptionist's desk to pay his bill in cash. The receptionist completes a copy of the bill and gives it to the patient as a receipt. However, the receptionist removes the other two copies of the document, as well as the cash, from the system. Since the receptionist has access to both the cash and the supporting record, she could remove both and go undetected **unless** you account for the prenumbered documents.

Thus, if you are using prenumbered documents and the numbering sequence is accounted for, removing a document would be promptly discovered. You can see from this example that the control value of prenumbered documents only works if you also account for the numbering sequence. Therefore, you need to keep all voided or altered documents in a file for reference purposes.

Internal Controls over the Cash Disbursement Function

The cash disbursement function actually begins when you place an order with a vendor or supplier. At that point, use a prenumbered document to substantiate your purchase. Then require the purchase to have approval by either a designated physician or the office manager.

When you mail a copy of the purchase order to the vendor, keep three copies: one in the purchase order file; the second for processing the invoice for payment; and the third for use as a receiving document. However, remove the quantity ordered from the third copy to require a physical count of the goods when they are received.

Once the receiving document substantiates the receipt of goods, a copy of the purchase order, the receiving document, and the invoice should be assembled as documentation to support the request for payment. At the point that the check is prepared and ready for signature, you should compare the documents as to the quantity ordered, etc., stamp the documents paid, and sign the checks. You should then give the checks to the receptionist for mailing and copies of the invoices with the supporting documents should be filed.

Once again, notice how many internal controls procedures are used in the cash disbursements cycle. First, the purchase orders are prenumbered and accounted for as described under the cash receipts cycle. Second, you use the authorization and approval process, both at the purchase order phase and the check signing phase. Then you use a comparison of documents, as well as stamping the documents "paid" to prevent any reprocessing. And last but not least, you use forward-processing for mailing checks to vendors.

Now that we have reviewed both the transaction and document flow for cash receipts and disbursements in Figures 7-2 and 7-3, examine Figures 7-4 and 7-5 to see where and how the controls occur in the process.

Now it is time for you to reflect on your own practice's policies and procedures used in these particular areas. Needless to say, each practice is different, and adapting these policies and procedures to your practice requires a great deal of thought.

Assessing Your Internal Controls

To begin this process, you must evaluate the current status of the policies and procedures used in your own practice. To help you in your assessment, we have prepared a list of internal control questions. These questions are broken down by functional area and we suggest that you read these questions carefully. If you answer "no" to any of the questions listed, there is room for improvement in the internal controls of your medical practice.

Internal Control Questions for Cash Receipts

Based on our earlier discussion, you should now be quite familiar with the controls necessary in the cash receipts function. To perform an assessment of your own practice, answer the following questions.

Does your medical practice:

_____ 1. Provide a written receipt at the point of service?

_____ 2. Require that a copy of the receipt be given to the patient?

_____ 3. Prepare daily cash deposits?

_____ 4. Compare the amount of cash deposited in the bank on a daily basis, to the amount shown as deposited in the accounting records?

_____ 5. Use one person to process cash and a separate individual to perform record-keeping responsibilities?

_____ 6. Restrict access to cash?

_____ 7. Restrict access to the accounting records?

_____ 8. Use only prenumbered receipts?

_____ 9. Separate the cash from the supporting documentation at the point of receipt?

_____10. Require preparation of a monthly bank reconcilement by someone other than those who process cash receipts and the accounting records that support the receipt of cash?

_____11. Bond all employees who have access to cash?

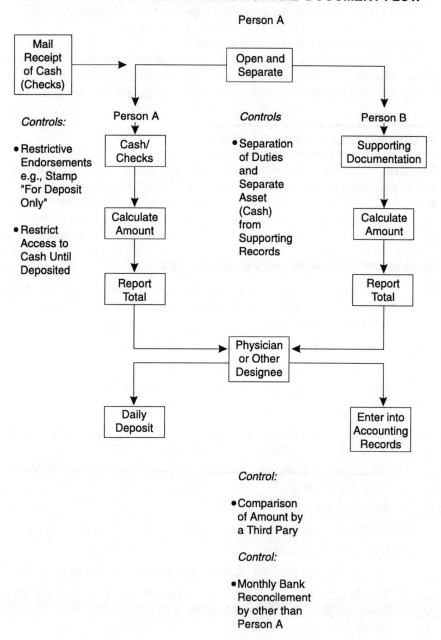

FIGURE 7-4
INTERNAL CONTROLS
CASH RECEIPTS CYCLE TRANSACTION AND DOCUMENT FLOW

FIGURE 7-5
CASH DISBURSEMENTS TRANSACTION AND DOCUMENT FLOW

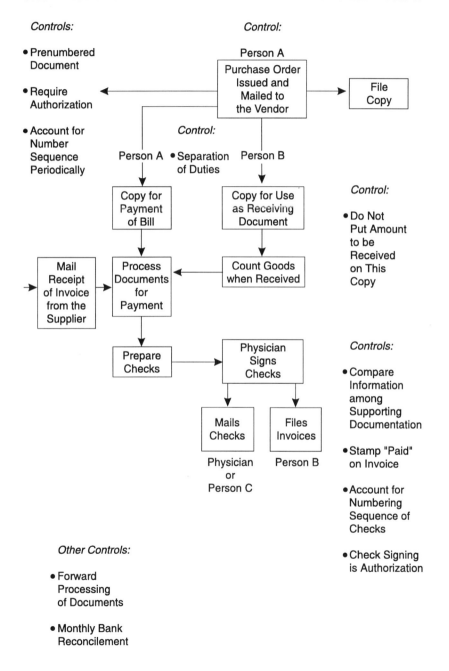

Controls:

- Prenumbered Document

- Require Authorization

- Account for Number Sequence Periodically

Control:

Person A

Purchase Order Issued and Mailed to the Vendor

File Copy

Control:

Person A • Separation of Duties   Person B

Copy for Payment of Bill

Copy for Use as Receiving Document

Mail Receipt of Invoice from the Supplier

Process Documents for Payment

Count Goods when Received

Control:

- Do Not Put Amount to be Received on This Copy

Prepare Checks

Physician Signs Checks

Controls:

- Compare Information among Supporting Documentation

Mails Checks

Files Invoices

- Stamp "Paid" on Invoice

Physician or Person C

Person B

- Account for Numbering Sequence of Checks

Other Controls:

- Forward Processing of Documents

- Monthly Bank Reconcilement

- Check Signing is Authorization

Internal Control Questions for Cash Disbursements

Similar to the cash receipts function, you now have a working knowledge of the cash disbursements function. To assess the status of your medical practice, answer the following questions.

Does your medical practice:

_____ 1. Use only prenumbered purchase orders?

_____ 2. Require approvals for purchase orders?

_____ 3. Require the use of bids when purchasing large quantities of merchandise, or purchasing medical or office equipment?

_____ 4. Remove the quantity ordered on the receiving copy of the purchase order?

_____ 5. Require the comparison of quantity, vendor, item number, etc., among the purchase order receiving document and invoice for every request for payment?

_____ 6. Require that the bills be paid by an employee who does not have access to the related asset?

_____ 7. Cancel all invoices when processed for payment?

_____ 8. Require disbursements by check only and require two signatures on checks over a prescribed amount?

_____ 9. Require that checks be mailed by an individual who has not been involved in the payment function?

_____10. Restrict access to unused, prenumbered checks?

Internal Control Questions for Payroll

Although the payroll function hasn't been described in detail in this chapter, we do not intend to underestimate its importance. It has not received separate attention thus far for two reasons: first, many medical practices use a payroll service for processing and preparing payroll; second, many of the internal control requirements for payroll disbursements are similar to that of the normal cash disbursements cycle. The major difference between payroll and other disbursements is the type of documentation required. While an invoice from a vendor is the standard document for a cash outlay in the normal cash disbursements cycle, a payroll time sheet or time card justifies payment of cash to an employee.

Because there are differences in the documentation for payroll disbursements, and assuming that payroll is not prepared by an outside payroll agency, you may wish to consider the following internal control questions concerning your payroll function.

Does your medical practice:

_____ 1. Provide some form of documentation and approval for the addition or deletion of employees from your work force?

_____ 2. Require the use of time cards or time sheets for all employees?

_____ 3. Indicate supervisory approval of the employee time card or sheet?

_____ 4. Periodically verify that the pay rates used to pay employees are the properly authorized amounts?

_____ 5. Verify gross and net pay?

_____ 6. Separate the individual who has responsibility for preparing the payroll checks from the individual who enters the information into the accounting system?

_____ 7. Require that checks be distributed to the employee by a physician?

_____ 8. Have checks signed by someone other than those who prepared them?

_____ 9. Have the checks signed by an individual other than the one authorized to hire personnel?

Other Internal Control Considerations

Many critical control questions occur in the cash receipts and disbursement areas. However, there are other types of transactions and internal control issues you need to evaluate. Therefore, you should also consider the following internal control questions.

Does your medical practice:

_____ 1. Maintain usage and inventory records for medical and office supplies?

_____ 2. Restrict access to supplies inventory?

_____ 3. Periodically reconcile the supply inventory on hand to the amount reported in the accounting records?

_____ 4. Require that patient refunds be supported by adequate documentation and approval by a physician?

_____ 5. Require that the write-off of a patient account be substantiated by appropriate documentation and be authorized by a designated physician?

_____ 6. Process only documents that have supporting information and approval?

_____ 7. Periodically review your accounting records, looking for unusual transactions?

_____ 8. Designate a specific individual in the medical practice responsible for authorization and approvals in the processing of transactions?

_____ 9. Periodically account for the numbering sequence in any prenumbered documents that are used?

_____10. Restrict and account for unused documents?

_____11. Restrict access to your accounting records?

_____12. Physically restrict access to your assets?

_____13. Reconcile the accounting information to the supporting documentation in the areas of receivables, inventory and property, and equipment?

_____14. Have established policies and procedures for job responsibilities of your employees?

_____15. Document these policies and procedures in writing?

_____16. Have an established accounting chart of accounts used for consistency in the medical practice?

It is obvious that there are a great number of policies and procedures that can be used to enhance the protection of your business assets. We are not advocating that each and every one of these be used in your practice since some of them may not be possible, given the size and scope of your medical practice.

However, we encourage you to periodically evaluate your policies and procedures to determine when and where additional controls are necessary or beneficial in protecting your business assets. In addition to asset protection, you should also determine that the documents recorded in the accounting records are properly processed.

Physician's Checklist

As a summary of this chapter, ask yourself the following questions. If you can answer "yes" to these questions, you have a good understanding of internal controls and the role they serve in protecting your business assets.

_____ 1. Do you understand why internal controls are necessary?

_____ 2. Does your practice actively use some of the internal control procedures described in this chapter?

_____ 3. Do you understand the characteristics that make certain policies and procedures useful in protecting your business assets?

_____ 4. Do you understand how even small medical practices, with a limited number of employees, can use certain policies and procedures to protect their assets?

_____ 5. Are you actively involved in the accounting function?

_____ 6. Has your practice assigned specific responsibility for authorizations and approvals of accounting transactions to a particular physician?

_____ 7. Do you understand the role you, as physician, play in making the environment conducive to internal controls?

_____ 8. Have you periodically evaluated your policies and procedures to determine where improvements can be made?

_____ 9. Do you understand how the lack of internal controls can hamper both the efficiency and effectiveness of your accounting system?

If you have answered "yes" to the questions above, you have an excellent understanding of the role of the internal control structure and how it applies to your business.

One of the issues discussed in this chapter was the internal control procedures that should govern acquisition of medical or office equipment. Another aspect of this purchasing decision is how the acquisition should be financed. The two choices are a purchase and the use of a lease arrangement. Chapter 8 considers the acquisition of property and equipment for your medical practice and helps you determine whether to lease or purchase the asset.

Questions and Answers

1. **My medical practice is quite small and I have only a few employees. How can I protect my business assets?**

   Protecting your business assets should be of prime concern to physicians. There are many policies and procedures that can be used even with a small number of employees to effectively provide some measure of control over the recording process and maintenance of the assets.

2. **What simple things can be done to help me protect my business assets?**

   Several easy things can be done to help you accomplish some measure of control over your cash receipts and cash disbursement cycle. Some of these are:

   - Use only prenumbered documents;
   - Mark all documents supporting disbursements "paid" as the check is prepared;
   - Compare documents supporting each transaction to determine that they agree as to critical information;
   - Use double signatures for checks over a certain dollar value;
   - Process information on a forward only basis (meaning do not return it to the individual who prepared the document);
   - Require documentation for all purchases;
   - Obtain bids for significant acquisitions of equipment;
   - Process transactions on a timely basis;
   - Restrict access to the assets;
   - Separate the asset from the accounting records that support it;
   - Bond employees who handle cash;
   - Actively manage your accounts receivable; and

- Periodically verify that the supporting accounting records match your actual assets used.

3. **Should I, as a physician, be involved in a plan designed to protect my assets?**

Never forget that the best internal control is your keen oversight of the financial and operating transactions in your practice. Many controls can be implemented, but your active oversight is absolutely essential to successfully protecting your assets.

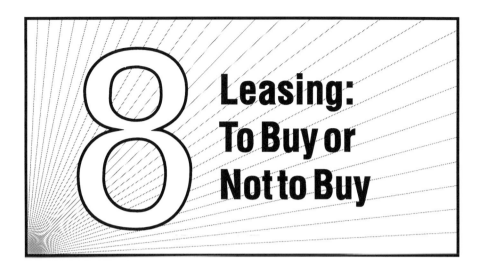

8. Leasing: To Buy or Not to Buy

There was no doubt that Dr. R. M. Lave's practice needed a new X-ray machine and Dr. Lave decided exactly which brand and model was best. Now the only question was whether to buy or lease the machine. In the meantime, he also looked at a new car and new office space and both of these decisions involved leasing questions as well.

Everything seemed so complicated. Leasing seemed to offer a tax advantage of being able to deduct the entire payment, but Dr. Lave's sense of old-fashioned values encouraged purchasing rather than renting. The dollar amounts involved were large and it appeared almost impossible to identify the cost differences for comparison purposes. Dr. Lave was particularly concerned about the impact that depreciation expense would have on the income of his practice and its corresponding income tax effect.

How do you make the right decisions with regard to purchasing or leasing? Is there a simple guideline to financial success or does each case need to be rigorously analyzed on an individual basis? Is it possible that depreciation expense can actually help the cash flow of the practice?

These are some of the primary questions addressed in this chapter. Leasing decisions can be extraordinarily complex. Leasing has a vocabulary of its own and leasing decisions often involve numerous benefits and costs that do not fit into simple formulas.

Nevertheless, a clear knowledge of the "big picture" and the basic vocabulary should enable you to make informed and successful leasing decisions for your medical practice. By the end of this chapter you should be able to understand the basic leasing terminology as well as the reasons for leasing on a conceptual basis, and to organize the costs and benefits of leasing into a numerical analysis that provides a dollar and cent answer to every leasing decision.

Specifically this chapter will address the following questions:

- What is an operating lease and what is a capital lease?
- How does depreciation affect taxes?
- How can I perform a simplified cost/benefit analysis?

Introduction and Overview of Leasing

Leasing is full of buzz-words. For starters, you may become confused over who is the lessor (the one who originally owns the asset) and who is the lessee (the one who rents the asset). Perhaps the problem arises from familiarity with the term renter and its similar sounding suffix with the term lessor.

One way to remember the distinction as you read this chapter and legal contracts, is to focus on the suffix "or" in the word less**or** and to think of the phrase "**or**iginally **o**wns." Thus the lessor originally owns the asset and is leasing it to the lessee.

To begin this overview of leasing, it's useful to distinguish between two intentions of leasing: operating leases and capital (or finance) leases.

Operating Leases: Leasing as "Temporary Rental"

In the case of *operating leases,* you lease when it is likely that you don't want the asset on a long-term basis (relative to the asset's useful life). Since you only plan on using the asset for a short period of time, you lease it to avoid the financial risk or the inconvenience of buying and then reselling the asset.

For example, if you own a growing medical practice, you might lease rather than purchase office space. One reason is because you may have long-term plans that call for a larger facility. In this case, it would be costly and inconvenient to purchase real estate now and then sell it in a few years when you move to a larger facility. Other reasons for renting are that you want to avoid the financial risk of real estate fluctuations, or you feel that you do not have the expertise to make a buying decision.

There are many other potential reasons to prefer an operating lease. For example, consider equipment that is subject to rapid technological change, such as the purchase of a new computer system or sophisticated medical equipment. You may need to change the equipment if the system doesn't perform properly or if it doesn't meet your needs. Thus, a lease may be the appropriate action in this case.

Thus, operating leases are used if you do not wish to enter the long-term financial commitment of a purchase or if rapid technological change is involved. Decisions on operating leases involve which asset to lease and how to negotiate terms, rather than whether to lease or to buy. The issues involved in operating lease decisions tend to be practice-specific issues rather than accounting and finance issues. For example, you may need to decide which equipment best meets your volume, size requirements, ease of operation, and so forth. In this chapter, we focus on the accounting, tax, and finance issues involved in lease versus buy decisions.

Leasing versus Buying: Capital (Finance) Leases

The alternative to an operating lease is a *capital* or finance lease. In a capital lease, you, the lessee, clearly are seeking a long-term commitment to use the asset—often the asset's entire useful life. The only decision is, in effect, a legal one: Should the asset be purchased or leased?

The example that we used earlier in the chapter was a capital lease. Dr. Lave knew which machine was best, expected to use the machine over most or all of its useful life, and only needed to decide whether to buy it or lease it.

When dealing with capital lease in a conceptual sense, the decision to buy or lease is best viewed as a question of paperwork. In other words, tax, legal, and accounting issues will dominate. These subjects will be detailed later in the chapter and a specific quantitative technique will be presented to help you make your decisions.

Sales and Leasebacks

As the name implies, a sale and leaseback occurs when you sell an asset that you currently own and then lease the asset back from the new owner.

Sale and leasebacks are usually regarded as a way to raise cash. The concept has been rarely used in managing small medical practices, but it is a concept that is worth a brief explanation.

For example, suppose that you own your office building. You can sell the real estate to an investor and simultaneously lease the facility back from the investor—maintaining continuous occupancy. You receive money from the sale and then make lease payments in the future. These transactions raise cash today and are, in effect, a method of borrowing money.

Alternatively, you could have borrowed money directly from a bank by obtaining a mortgage on the facility. Common reasons to use a sale and leaseback, rather than borrow the money directly, are to obtain better interest rates or tax considerations. For example, if you currently have accounting losses, you may find it useful from a tax perspective to sell and leaseback real estate and equipment that was previously purchased.

A final issue worth noting is protecting your assets from liability risks, such as legal actions. As discussed in Chapter 2, many medical practices seek forms of business organization that reduce taxes and provide increased protection from liability. You may find it useful to own an asset, such as a building or equipment, through one business and use it in your medical practice. Leasing can be an ideal tool. If your medical practice already owns the asset, you might explore the sale and leaseback option as a method of improving your tax and legal situation.

Depreciation and Leasing from a Tax Perspective

In this section, we focus on the accounting and tax perspectives of leasing versus buying, rather than issues such as convenience and maintenance.

The decision to lease rather than buy affects the paperwork in several important ways. The most important issue is who gets to depreciate the asset for tax purposes.

The next few subsections get a little complicated, so it might help to know what we are going to do. In short, we are going to explain that depreciation expense is a good thing. These subsections fully explain two points:

1. Depreciation expense offers a tax benefit to those who own assets; and

2. Assets should often be owned by those in high tax brackets rather than those in low tax brackets.

First, we detail the tax effects of depreciation. Understanding these tax effects is crucial to performing cost/benefit analyses in subsequent sections.

Depreciation

Depreciation is the accounting and tax recognition of the decline in the value of an asset. Depreciation expense is an accounting number, not a cash flow. As discussed in Chapter 5, depreciation is the regular "writing off" or expensing of the value of an asset downward from its purchase price. Thus, accountants view depreciation as an expense.

However, in this chapter we need to view depreciation as an opportunity to improve cash flow! Generally, each dollar of depreciation reduces taxable income by one dollar and therefore reduces taxes. For example, a taxpayer in a 40 percent tax bracket can reduce taxes by $0.40 for each dollar of depreciation. Thus, even though depreciation is an expense, it serves to reduce the expected cash outflow by paying less in income taxes. If you own an asset, you can use depreciation to create a cash flow in the form of reduced income taxes.

In most cases, tax laws allow accountants to claim a greater decline in the value of an asset in the asset's early years than actually occurs. This accelerated depreciation can be an important tax advantage.

For example, consider real estate, such as an office building, that you just purchased for $1,000,000. We picked $1,000,000 because it is a nice round number even though obviously the typical medical practice would require a smaller building. Also, as previously discussed, a medical professional typically would own an office building in a separate business organization from his or her medical practice.

In most real estate markets and at most points in time, few people would expect the price of the office building to decline rapidly in value. Many people would predict that it could decline and sometimes does, but few people would expect the decline and forecast the decline as the most likely event. Nevertheless, tax laws allow the purchase price of the building to be depreciated, thereby reducing the value of the building (not including the value of the land).

Computing exactly how much depreciation can be taken in each year of an asset's life is complicated and the rules change regularly. For simplicity, let's assume that the rules allow the above $1,000,000 office building to be depreciated by $30,000 in the first year, $32,000 in the second year, $32,000 in the third year, and continuing until the entire $1,000,000 has been depreciated over a total of 32 years. Finally, let's assume that you, the owner, are in a 40 percent tax bracket (including Federal, state, and local income tax rates) with plenty of taxable income.

As owner of the building, you can lower your taxable income by $30,000 in the first year by claiming the depreciation as an expense. This results in reducing your income taxes by $12,000 (found by multiplying the depreciation amount by the tax rate, i.e., $30,000 x .40). Remember, you haven't really lost $30,000 because in most cases the value of the property is actually holding constant or perhaps even rising. Instead, you use the depreciation to decrease your income taxes.

You can continue to lower your income tax bills during the subsequent years by claiming the allowable depreciation expense, even if the true market value of the office building is rising. Thus, throughout the next 32 years, you can avoid paying income taxes on $1,000,000 of income even though it is quite possible that your $1,000,000 investment in the office building has actually risen in market value. This $1,000,000 of depreciation expense decreases income taxes totaling $400,000 if you remain in a 40 percent tax bracket.

Thus, a primary benefit of owning an asset is the ability to depreciate the asset. This tax benefit needs to be included in a cost/benefit analysis, detailed later in the chapter.

Eventually, you will probably sell the building and at that time you will probably have to pay taxes on the gain from the sale—in effect, paying tax on all of the depreciation that was written off in the previous years. All of those years of depreciation have reduced the value of the asset to zero in your tax and accounting records. Therefore, your basis is zero and any amount received results in a gain.

However, the timing of receiving the tax break now but paying taxes on a gain later creates a financial benefit. This timing benefit is detailed below.

The Time Value Benefit of Depreciation

As the owner in the above example, you pay income taxes on the gain when the building is sold because of the depreciation deductions that were claimed throughout the years. But here is the key: you received reduced taxes in the early years and then paid taxes on the gain later. The advantage of accelerated depreciation is that it produces tax savings today but doesn't cause added taxes until the future. This serves as an interest-free loan from the government.

In the previous example, we assumed you were in a 40 percent tax bracket. Therefore, the full depreciation of the building over 32 years resulted in $400,000 of reduced taxes!

Let's assume for simplicity, that you received $12,500 in tax breaks each year for 32 years and placed these funds in a bank account earning 6 percent interest after taxes. We selected an after-tax interest rate of 6 percent purely for simplicity. Including this interest (after taxes) the bank account would be worth $1,136,122 at the end of the thirty-second year, reflecting the final value of your tax savings created by the depreciation expense!

Now let's assume that after 32 years you sell the building for $1,500,000. In the year that the building is sold, you would probably have to pay significant taxes on the gain since the accounting book value or "tax basis" of the asset has been depreciated to a value of zero. You would have to pay taxes on both the $500,000 gain and the $1,000,000 of recaptured depreciation.

However, 40 percent taxes on the $1,000,000 of recaptured depreciation is $400,000 and is far short of the $1,136,122 of tax savings obtained throughout the years, when you consider the time value of money. Thus, as an owner you can receive a substantial tax advantage by saving taxes in the early years, even if taxes must eventually be paid when the asset is sold.

The tax advantage discussed above is even more impressive if you can avoid paying full taxes when the building is sold. For example, capital gains tax benefits and careful estate planning can reduce the taxes due on the sale. In some cases the tax liability on the sale can be delayed.

Further, you might be able to time the transactions so that the depreciation deduction is declared in years of high income and high tax rates. When tax brackets are highest, tax breaks create the highest cash savings. Conversely, if you sell the asset near retirement, the asset can be sold and the gain declared when you have less income and/or reside in a state with little or no income taxes, such that the taxes paid on the sale are reduced.

Careful estate planning can also be used to reduce or even eliminate taxes on the gain. The strategies that can be used to postpone or avoid taxes are complex, numerous, and constantly changing. Obviously, you need to regularly consult a qualified professional.

Remember, depreciation is an accounting number, not a cash expense. Depreciation creates cash savings through tax savings. These savings can be substantial when the time value of money is included and they must be included in an accurate cost/benefit analysis.

The Tax Rate Differentials as the Key

The above discussion cited the tax advantages of depreciation in detail. At first, it appears to encourage asset ownership from a tax perspective. The message seems to be that the tax advantages of depreciation should encourage you to own, rather than lease, assets.

However, we will now show you that the best tax advantages occur when the people who own the asset are those in the highest tax bracket. Thus, the same leasing deal may be beneficial for some but not for all.

In fact, one of the primary motivations for leasing can be to allow the asset to be owned by people in high tax brackets and leased to people in lower tax brackets. This situation relies upon the idea that the owner will pass much of the tax savings along to the lessee, in the form of lower lease payments.

Let's return to the previous example of a $1,000,000 office building that can be depreciated over the next 32 years. Consider what would have happened if you had only been in a 20 percent combined tax bracket. Using a 20 percent tax rate, claiming $30,000 of depreciation expense reduces taxes by only $6,000. This contrasts with $12,000 of tax savings enjoyed if you are in a 40 percent tax bracket. Over the 32 years, the building's full depreciation of $1,000,000 would reduce taxes by only $200,000 if you are in a 20 percent tax bracket compared to $400,000 if you are a 40 percent (high) income tax bracket payer.

Thus, if you are a medical professional just getting started and have low income, you might find yourself in a low tax bracket where the tax advantages of asset ownership would be largely wasted. Worse yet, imagine depreciating an asset through years of low taxes and correspondingly low tax savings only to sell the asset years later when income is high and then having to pay enormous taxes on the gain.

One solution to a medical professional's dilemma would be to lease the asset from a firm or person in a very high tax bracket who would benefit greatly from tax breaks.

Remember, leasing allows one person or business organization to use an asset (the lessee) while another person or business organization owns the asset (the lessor). For tax reasons, leasing is often used to allow the person in the highest tax bracket to receive tax breaks rather than having them partially or fully wasted by a person in a low tax bracket or with losses.

However, the key to tax-motivated leasing is that the lessor must pass some of these tax benefits to the lessee in the form of reduced lease payments. Lessors can be forced to pass along some of these benefits through competition. Alternatively, the lessor may be related to the lessee such as when a medical professional owns the asset through one business organization and leases it to his or her medical practice.

One of the clearest examples is the case of a not-for-profit organization that pays no income taxes. Such organizations derive no tax benefit from depreciation. Therefore, it makes sense for them to lease their assets from those who receive the benefits from depreciation and pass those benefits along to the lessee.

In a competitive or negotiated situation, the key is to decide to buy or lease based upon the idea that the person in the highest tax bracket should claim depreciation. This permits the highest total tax savings which presumably can be shared by the lessor and lessee. Often, leasing can help facilitate this overall tax benefit. However, as discussed later in the chapter, the lessee can sometimes claim the depreciation rather than the lessor.

One word of caution before we proceed. The virtues of depreciation cited above depended upon two factors. First, the example above had depreciation for an asset with a long life, held for a long period of time, so that the time value of money produced an enormous effect. In contrast, assets with shorter lives produce substantially lower tax advantages.

Second, the example relied upon the idea that the asset was being depreciated to accounting book values, which were lower than the market value of the asset. Thus, the owner was allowed to claim an expense that was not occurring in an economic sense. The more quickly an asset can be depreciated and the longer term the true life of the asset, the greater the tax advantage.

Now that you understand the importance of depreciation and one of the conceptual reasons for deciding to lease or buy, how do you actually make a decision regarding a specific lease or buy alternative? The following discussion will help you make these decisions.

A Simplified Cost/Benefit Analysis

The purpose of this section is to detail an accurate procedure for analyzing the lease versus buy decision when acquiring an asset.

The important words in the above sentence are accurate procedure and analyzing. There is a tendency for people to want a general recommendation like "you should always lease your assets because . . . ." However, you must realize that each specific case is different. To receive the right answer to the lease versus buy question, you or your accountant must apply the procedure described in this chapter to each set of facts.

When you read the remainder of this chapter, your initial reaction will probably be "that is why I have an accountant." We urge you to reconsider that philosophy.

Although this process may appear foreign and difficult to you, it is a necessary requirement if you are to make correct purchasing decisions. Even if you ask your accountant to perform the "number crunching" aspects, you still need to understand what is involved in the process to make informed decisions.

The procedure used in this discussion produces a bottom line amount that represents the total incremental cost of each alternative in today's dollars. Therefore, the lease versus buy decision is reduced to selecting the lower cost alternative. We will then demonstrate the process through the hypothetical acquisition of a machine.

The previous section detailed one of the trickiest issues in the analysis—depreciation. This section will build the tax advantage of depreciation into the analysis.

The analysis presented in this section involves four steps:

1. Compile the costs of each alternative;

2. Place the costs and other information into the figure provided;

3. Total the costs for each time period using the cash flow formula; and

4. Combine the cash flows into a single value for each alternative by discounting them for the time value of money and summing them.

The whole procedure appears complicated at first, so it might be useful to periodically refer back to the above four steps to help you remember where you are in the process. Let's start by looking at the figure that will be used.

A Figure for Summarizing Costs

Figure 8-1 provides spaces for you to input the relevant factors of either owning or leasing an asset. These factors are listed in the various column headings, while each year of the asset life and its effects is shown by rows. To save space, the figure shows only three

FIGURE 8-1
THE CASH FLOWS OF AN ASSET

Time Period	(1) Taxable Cash Flow	(2) Depreciation Expense	(3) Tax Rate	(4) Nontaxable Cash Flow		(5) Total Cash Flow for Period
0	___	___	___	___	=>	___
1	___	___	___	___	=>	___
2	___	___	___	___	=>	___
3	___	___	___	___	=>	___
			Bottom Line Result			___

time periods. Obviously, in practice the figure contains the time periods for the entire life of the alternative.

The best way to utilize this analysis is to place it on a computerized spreadsheet. By doing this, the math can be done quickly and accurately. Further, the inputs can be efficiently changed as new information becomes available, or for new alternatives. Finally, you can vary the inputs to test the effect of various assumptions on the decision. This is known as "what if," or sensitivity analysis. However, a computerized spreadsheet is not necessary and the analysis shown in this book will be done without one.

In summary, you should compute an analysis as shown in Figure 8-1 for each lease or buy alternative. The idea is to fill in the first four columns of blanks using the specific information relevant to each asset acquisition. Then use a formula to compute the final (fifth) column and total the final column. Finally, you take into account the time value of money by collapsing the fifth column into one final figure, the "Bottom Line Result." The alternative with the better bottom line result should be selected.

Let's examine the key elements:

1. The time period selected does not have to be years. In other words, time period one does not have to mean the first year. The figure could be based upon quarters or even months. The decision should be based upon the life of the asset and the precision of the costs being included. An asset with a long life, such as a building, should be analyzed in years. Equipment with a life of three to five years should be measured in quarters if the costs are accurately estimated. Time period 0 refers to immediate figures, such as a purchase price or down payment, and should be included in the first line.

2. For most decisions, almost all of the input figures are costs and should be entered as negative numbers because they are cash outflows. However, some cash inflows might be included, such as the proceeds from selling an asset (e.g., a car) when it is no longer needed. Cash inflows should be included as positive numbers.

3.   There are three main types of inputs: taxable cash flows (column 1), depreciation (column 2), and nontaxable cash flows (column 4). All benefits and costs should fall into one of these three categories. When a taxable cash flow (column 1) is an outflow, it is called *tax deductible.*

4.   The tax rate (column 3) is the sum of federal, state, and local income tax rates. This is allowed to change over time if you think that either the tax rates or your income tax bracket will change significantly. The tax rates used should correspond to the business organization reporting the transaction.

The analysis is performed by completing Figure 8-1 for each alternative. The best alternative is the one with the lowest final cost.

Initial, Operations, and Termination Cash Flows

The analysis can be simplified by viewing the cash flows in three stages of time: initial, operating, and termination. Most of the cash flows from initiating the alternative, such as a purchase price or down payment, occur immediately—at time period zero. Similar types of cash flows occur throughout each alternative's life—the operating stage. These cash flows would include regular payments, regular cash expenses, and depreciation. Finally, there are often special cash flows that occur in the last time period, such as the sale of the asset or the closing of the lease.

We will now consider the first step of completing the analysis for the "buying alternative"—the decision to buy an asset. Remember, we are detailing the issues used to decide which is more beneficial: buying or leasing.

The Cash Flows of Buying

The first step in the analysis process is to collect the data for each alternative. The procedure is simple: collect all of the costs and (perhaps with help from your accountant) divide the costs into those that are tax deductible because they are a current period operating expense (referred to as taxable) and those that are not tax deductible (referred to as nontaxable).

There is one very important but tricky point: you include only those figures that are different for the alternatives. In other words, any amount that is the same in both alternatives, can be ignored. This can simplify the analysis considerably.

As an example, let's consider the purchase of an automobile. The moment the car is purchased, you incur a number of costs. At this point, you need to focus on cash outlays. For example, the purchase may require a $1,000 down payment, $100 in loan fees, and $300 in licensing and other fees. Thus, the total required down payment is $1,400.

First, consider the figures unique to this alternative. If you must pay the $300 in licensing and other fees even if you lease the vehicle, then it is not necessary to include the $300 in either analysis. It won't hurt to include the $300 figure in both analyses but it is a waste of time.

Second, look at cash flows from your pocket. If a loan is used, do not include the costs that are paid using the loan money. The costs paid with the loan money are included when you include the cost of repaying the loan. Ask yourself the question: does this cost require me to write a check?

Let's start with the cash flows during the initial stage. Your accountant tells you that the $100 loan fee is tax deductible as an operating expense of the business in the period in which it is paid and the $1,000 down payment is not. For simplicity, we'll assume that these are the only cash flows that occur when the car is purchased—the initial stage.

Since you plan on owning the car for three years and because the figures can be estimated accurately, you decide to base the analysis on 12 quarters rather than three years.

Next, the cash expenses for each quarter are identified for the operating stage. These cash flows include loan payments and any expenses that would not be incurred if the car were leased. These costs need to be separated into the tax deductible and nontaxable portions. For example, each loan payment can be divided into a tax deductible component (the interest) and a nontaxable component (the principal). The interest component is the expense you pay for receiving the loan. The principal is the cash you spend to repay the loan and reduce your indebtedness.

The depreciation expense for each quarter must also be calculated to include the tax savings discussed in the previous section.

Finally, the cash flows from selling the car and repaying the loan should be included in the final quarter—the termination stage. The proceeds from selling the car should be divided into a nontaxable portion (the basis or accounting book value of the car) and the taxable portion (any profit or loss relative to the accounting value of the car). The funds used to repay the loan might be divided between the nontaxable portion (the principal payoff) and a tax deductible portion, such as a loan payoff or recording fee.

Figure 8-2 illustrates the above discussion and provides numbers to demonstrate an analysis.

Obviously, the input data required can be numerous for significant and long-range decisions. The analysis provided above is significantly simplified. To be completely accurate, it might also be useful to recognize the difference between when expenses are paid and when they can be deducted for tax purposes, such as insurance costs. To be realistic, you must realize that many of the figures are rough estimates (e.g., the price at which the car can be sold at the end of three years).

Nevertheless, an accurate analysis might require the collection of all costs and the division of those costs, within each time period, into those that can, and cannot, be deducted for tax purposes.

In the above discussion, we illustrated the data for the financial analysis of buying. Next, we illustrate the data for the leasing alternative.

The Cash Flows of Leasing

The leasing alternative starts with the same analysis—in this case Figure 8-1. We repeat the process of identifying all cash outlays that are unique to leasing the asset and dividing

FIGURE 8-2
THE CASH FLOWS OF BUYING A CAR

Time Period	(1) Taxable Cash Flow	(2) Depreciation Expense	(3) Tax Rate	(4) Nontaxable Cash Flow		(5) Total Cash Flow for Period
0	−100	0	.36	−1,000	=>	_____
1	−400	−2,000	.36	−1,600	=>	_____
2	−380	−1,800	.36	−1,620	=>	_____
3	−360	−1,600	.36	−1,640	=>	_____
		[Periods 4 through 11 Not Shown]				
12	8,000	0	.36	−6,000	=>	_____
				Bottom Line Result		_____

them based upon their tax treatment. Again for simplicity, our collection of these cash flows is organized into three stages: initial, operating, and termination.

One of the essential elements of leasing is that the lessee may be able to claim depreciation in some circumstances. However, they cannot deduct both depreciation and the lease payment. For our example, we will assume that the full lease payment is deductible but that the depreciation is claimed by the lessor (i.e., the car company).

The cash flows of the initial stage are often easier for leasing. In our example, the lease requires no down payment other than the $300 fee for licensing and other fees. However, as discussed previously, this $300 payment must be made whether the car is purchased or leased. Therefore, it is not unique to the leasing alternative and will not be included in the analysis.

The leasing payments throughout the operating phase are also straightforward. The only cash flow is a $500 monthly lease payment that is fully tax deductible.

Finally, the termination phase involves those cash flows unique to leasing that will occur when the contract ends in the twelfth quarter. Often an automotive lease will call for cash flows at the end of the leasing period based upon mileage and condition of the car. For simplicity, we will assume that no further costs are anticipated.

All of these cash flows are placed in a table for leasing cash flows as demonstrated in Figure 8-3.

The Total Cash Flow Column

Now that the costs have been included for each analysis, the final (fifth) column must be computed for each alternative and for each time period. The total cash flow figure is derived from the figures in columns one through four. The formula for computing the total figure may be solved by hand or programmed into a computerized spreadsheet.

FIGURE 8-3
THE CASH FLOWS OF LEASING A CAR

Time Period	(1) Taxable Cash Flow	(2) Depreciation Expense	(3) Tax Rate	(4) Nontaxable Cash Flow		(5) Total Cash Flow for Period
0	0	0	.36	0	=>	_____
1	-1,500	0	.36	0	=>	_____
2	-1,500	0	.36	0	=>	_____
3	-1,500	0	.36	0	=>	_____
		[Periods 4 through 11 Not Shown]				
12	-1,500	0	.36	0	=>	_____
				Bottom Line Result		======

In order to abbreviate the names for the values in each of the columns, let's define TCF as the value from the first column (the taxable cash flow), DE as the value from the second column, NTCF as the value from the fourth column, and ACF as the value from the fifth column, and so forth. Be sure that the tax rate, TR, is expressed as a decimal (e.g., 0.36) rather than as a percentage (e.g., 36.0). Given these abbreviated names, the formula for the aggregate cash flow, ACF, in the fifth column is:

$$ACF = [(TCF + DE) * (1 - TR)] + (-DE) + NTCF$$

The logic of the formula is that the terms inside the brackets form after-tax incremental expense; depreciation is added back since it is a noncash expense; and nontaxable cash flows are added.

For example, the first time period of the purchase (buying) example (Figure 8-2) has the following values:

TCF   = Taxable Cash Flow = -400;
DE   = Depreciation Expense = -2,000;
TR   = Tax Rate = .36; and
NTCF = Nontaxable Cash Flow = -1,600

Inserting these values into the formula for ACF (the aggregate cash flow for the time period),

$$ACF = [(TCF + DE) * (1 - TR)] + (-DE) + NTCF$$

produces:

$$ACF = [(-400 + -2,000) * .64] + 2,000 -1,600$$

which reduces to:

$$ACF = -1,536 + 2,000 - 1,600 = -1,136$$

Note that even though Figure 8-2 indicates that $1,600 will be spent on a nontaxable basis and $400 will be spent on a taxable basis, the total cash outflow for the period is only $1,136. This is due to the depreciation tax effect and the tax savings from the $400 tax deductible expense.

The above process should be used to produce a figure for each row of column 5 corresponding to each time period. Next, we begin the process of combining the fifth column into a single Bottom Line Result.

Selecting a Discount Rate

At first it might be tempting to simply total the figures from the fifth column of aggregate cash flows into an final total cost figure. However, it is essential to account for the time value of money. In other words, we must take into account the current interest rate in order to covert future cash flows into present day values. There can be a big difference between paying $1,000 today and paying $1,000 in 5 or 10 years.

The *discount rate* is the interest rate used to adjust a future cash flow to its value in today's dollars—its present value. For example, suppose that by purchasing rather than leasing equipment, you find that you will be able to sell the equipment at the end of four years for $5,000. Obviously, this is a valuable benefit that needs to be included in the analysis. However, the hope of receiving $5,000 four years from today is worth less than $5,000 in today's dollars, especially if inflation and interest rates are high.

A discount rate can be used to adjust or discount the $5,000 into a lower figure in terms of today's dollars—a present value. This discussion walks you through the process of adjusting the cash flows from each period into a single time-adjusted value.

A future cash flow is adjusted backwards toward the present time one period when it is divided by the quantity *1 + r,* where *r* is the discount rate expressed as a decimal quantity.

For example, if the discount rate is 10 percent, then the discount rate is 0.10 expressed as a decimal value and a cash flow can be discounted for one period by dividing the cash flow by 1 + 0.10 or simply 1.10. In the example above, we assumed the receipt of $5,000 in four years. This $5,000 can be discounted back to year three by dividing the $5,000 by 1.10. The resulting figure ($4,545.45) is the value of the cash flow in terms of dollars in year three.

By dividing the $4,545.45 again by 1.10 the value can be moved backwards another year to year two, producing a year two value of $4,132.23. If the resulting quantity is divided by 1.10 two more times, then the value is moved backwards another two years to the current time, year 0.

The final figure, $3,415.07, is known as the *present value.* It is viewed as the equivalent value in today's dollars of receiving $5,000 four years later, given a discount rate of 10 percent. When all cash flows within a decision have been moved backward or discounted into present values, they can be accurately compared and analyzed.

There has been tremendous debate over the selection of an appropriate discount rate. Volumes of material have been written on how to determine an appropriate rate. The issue can become quite complicated.

As a simple method, we suggest selecting a discount rate using current interest rates. You should probably use an interest rate somewhere between short-term certificate of deposit (CD) rates offered at local banks and the current 30-year fixed rate mortgage rates. For short, low risk decisions, the discount rate should be closer to the short-term CD rate (i.e., a one-year certificate of deposit). For longer-term and riskier decisions, a rate near the current fixed rate mortgage rate would be more appropriate. These rates can readily be found in most newspapers.

The discount rate selected can also depend upon your financial circumstances. The appropriate interest rate is often best measured as the interest rate that you would pay or receive on the money involved.

If you have surplus cash, you should select a discount rate equal to the interest rate associated with your excess cash. If you had extra money, where would you invest the money and what rate would you receive? Would you use extra money to pay off a loan or would you make an investment? What would be the approximate interest rate that you would save or earn on these extra funds?

If you need cash, you should select a discount rate equal to the interest rate you would have to pay to obtain cash. If extra money were needed, where would you obtain it (e.g., a bank loan, a home equity line of credit, or savings)? What would be the approximate interest rate that would be paid or lost on these needed funds?

If there is a clear source or use of extra funds, then the rate offered on these funds would probably be the best discount rate to use. However, we suggest that you not spend time worrying about selecting the appropriate discount rate. Rather, you should focus on the more important issues, such as projecting cash flows accurately.

You must recognize that the cost/benefit analysis detailed in this section relies upon projections of cash flows that probably contain significant error. The old saying: "garbage in, garbage out" applies here. For example, we discussed a projection of receiving $5,000 from the sale of the asset after four years. In practice, this $5,000 figure would typically be a very rough approximation. Hence, it doesn't pay to spend too much time worrying about an exact discount rate.

Once a discount rate has been determined, the cash flows in the fifth column (the total or aggregate cash flow for each time period) need to be discounted and summed. Many people have experience in performing this procedure and many computerized spreadsheets will do the math for you. If you wish to see how the mathematics work, see the Appendix.

Comparing the Present Values

The final step in the process is the easiest and answers your lease versus buy decision! You simply compare the final results of each alternative and select the method with the best Bottom Line Result. If one alternative is positive and one is negative, the positive one should be selected. Typically, both alternatives will have negative values. Therefore, the value closest to zero should be selected.

The Bottom Line Result measures the total costs that are unique to the given alternative. The results do not tell you the value of the alternative to the firm since benefits and costs shared by the alternatives are omitted. However, the difference between the results is the value added to your medical practice by selecting the better, rather than the worse, alternative.

An Example Analysis

The above procedure has been fully explained from start to finish. It may appear cumbersome the first time through. This section will demonstrate the procedure by introducing a relatively simple lease versus buy decision. As we go through the procedure, we'll attempt to emphasize the aspects that you might find troublesome.

The Facts

Our example is a piece of equipment from FM Corp. that costs $100,000, or can be leased for two years at a monthly lease payment of $4,000 with no money down and no further cash flows at the end of the lease. The leasing contract does not call for FM Corp. to provide maintenance and repairs. Whether you buy or lease the machine, a maintenance contract can be purchased for $250 per month.

Your business organization is in a 35 percent total tax bracket including Federal, state, and local income taxes.

In a typical decision, there would be additional information. For example, you might plan on using the equipment 10 times per day, 200 days per year with $100 billing per use. However, only a portion of the billable amount will probably be collected. Each usage costs $12 in other materials.

However, the cash inflows discussed in the above paragraph occur regardless of whether the machine is purchased or leased. Therefore, they can be omitted from the analysis. For that reason, the $250 maintenance contract can also be omitted.

At the end of two years, the medical practice expects to obtain more sophisticated equipment. It is expected that the machine could be sold for $20,000, if it has been purchased, or it could be returned to the lessor at no cost, if it has been leased.

The $100,000 purchase can be financed with a $95,000 loan, requiring $5,000 down and 24 monthly payments of $4,340.05 each. The machine can be depreciated at the rate of $12,500 per quarter. We use this depreciation figure for simplicity even though it is unrelated to current tax laws.

Although the problem involves 24 months, it is probably useful to simplify the analysis by reducing the analysis to eight quarters, especially if a computerized spreadsheet is not being used. This saves time and potential for error.

The Cash Flows of Buying

You must remember that the analysis should only include those cash flows unique to the alternative. Thus, we seek to identify and place in the figure, those cash flows that will occur only if the machine is purchased rather than leased.

In order to organize the process, we will work through the cash flows in the three stages previously given: initial, operating, and termination.

First, the initial stage, time zero, is simple. There is a $5,000 nontax deductible down payment.

The operational stage is more complex because the monthly payments must be divided into interest portions that are tax deductible and principal portions that are not. If you cannot or do not want to do this, the loan company or your accountant can provide the information. In essence, it requires a loan amortization chart that shows the portion of the payment applied to interest (and therefore taxable or tax deductible) and the portion of the payment that reduces the loan balance (the nontaxable portion). Figure 8-5 reflects the partitioning. Additionally, Figure 8-5 reflects the depreciation.

Finally, the terminal stage involves receiving $20,000 upon subsequent sale of the equipment. The complexity of this event is dividing the sales proceeds between the nontaxable portion (the asset's book value) and the taxable portion (the profit or loss on the sale relative to the book value). In our example, the asset has been depreciated to a book value of zero by the end of the final quarter and therefore the entire $20,000 selling price results in a taxable gain.

The above computations complete columns one through four for Figure 8-4 for the buying or purchase decision. To complete Figure 8-4, you use the formula for column five and then discount column five to the Bottom Line Result.

Next, we do the easier part: the leasing analysis. When that is completed, the results can be compared and you can make your decision.

The Cash Flow of Leasing

The cash flows of leasing are extremely simple in this example. Once again, we need to consider those cash flows that will occur only if we lease the equipment. In this case, the relevant cash flow is the $4,000 monthly lease payment and it is fully taxable (or since it is an expense, it is tax deductible). Thus, $12,000 per quarter is included as a taxable cash flow. There is no depreciation allowed and no down payments or final cash flows. Accordingly, Figure 8-5 merely reflects the lease payments.

Next, we select a discount rate, compute the results, and compare them.

Selecting a Discount Rate

Finally, with the purchase of equipment, extra cash flow is required, both to meet the down payment and the higher monthly payments. Ultimately, these cash requirements restrict the practice's ability to repay its bank loan with interest of 12 percent. Accordingly, 12 percent is selected as the annual interest rate. Since our analysis is quarterly, we divide 12 percent by 4 to obtain the 3 percent quarterly interest rate.

Making the Decision

The fifth columns of the two alternatives (Figures 8-4 and 8-5) are computed using the formula and discounted using the 12 percent interest rate. This step is shown in Figure 8-6. The two columns entitled "Total Cash Flow for Period" are taken from completed versions of the fifth column of Figures 8-4 and 8-5.

FIGURE 8-4
THE CASH FLOW OF BUYING THE X-RAY MACHINE

Time Period	(1) Taxable Cash Flow	(2) Depreciation Expense	(3) Tax Rate	(4) Nontaxable Cash Flow		(5) Total Cash Flow for Period
0	–0		.35	–5,000	=>	_____
1	–2,056	–12,500	.35	–10,964	=>	_____
2	–1,807	–12,500	.35	–11,213	=>	_____
3	–1,553	–12,500	.35	–11,467	=>	_____
4	–1,293	–12,500	.35	–11,727	=>	_____
5	–1,027	–12,500	.35	–11,993	=>	_____
6	–755	–12,500	.35	–12,265	=>	_____
7	–477	–12,500	.35	–12,543	=>	_____
8	19,807	–12,500	.35	–12,827	=>	_____
			Bottom Line Result			_____

The columns entitled "Discounted Cumulative Sum" show the subtotals obtained from performing the discounting shortcut. Recall that the shortcut discounting method starts with the figure from the last time period, discounts the sum for one time period using the sum of one plus the given interest rate (3 percent per quarter), and adds it to the current quarter. The figures move upward from the last row to the first row and show these subtotals.

The final discounted cumulative sum (taken from the first row) is the Bottom Line Result. Our analysis shows that the leasing alternative has a Bottom Line Result of –$54,754 while purchasing has a Bottom Line Result of –$52,509. Thus, purchasing has a lower total cost, in present value dollars, of $2,245. In this situation, the medical practice is better off purchasing than leasing.

The process may appear cumbersome, but it has an important point. The higher annual costs of buying the machine are worthwhile, given that you would own the machine and you could sell it for $20,000 when the medical practice was finished with it. When the time value of money is taken into account, paying the $5,000 down payment today and waiting eight quarters to receive the $20,000 made purchasing the better alternative.

The depreciation didn't produce a big tax savings in a present value sense, since the equipment was only used for two years.

Remember, since cash flows common to each alternative are best omitted from the analysis, the Bottom Line Results do not necessarily measure the total costs of each alternative. Rather, the difference between the Bottom Line Results reflects the advantage of the lower cost alternative over the higher cost alternative. Thus in our example,

FIGURE 8-5
THE CASH FLOW OF LEASING THE X-RAY MACHINE

Time Period	(1) Taxable Cash Flow	(2) Depreciation Expense	(3) Tax Rate	(4) Nontaxable Cash Flow		(5) Total Cash Flow for Period
0	–0	0	.35	0	=>	_____
1	–12,000	0	.35	0	=>	_____
2	–12,000	0	.35	0	=>	_____
3	–12,000	0	.35	0	=>	_____
4	–12,000	0	.35	0	=>	_____
5	–12,000	0	.35	0	=>	_____
6	–12,000	0	.35	0	=>	_____
7	–12,000	0	.35	0	=>	_____
8	–12,000	0	.35	0	=>	_____
				Bottom Line Result		_____

FIGURE 8-6
LEASING VERSUS BUYING THE X-RAY MACHINE

Time Period	BUYING Total Cash Flow for Period	BUYING Discounted Cumulative Sum	LEASING Total Cash Flow for Period	LEASING Discounted Cumulative Sum
0	–$5,000	–$52,509	0	–$54,754
1	–$7,926	–$48,934	–$7,800	–$56,396
2	–$8,013	–$42,239	–$7,800	–$50,054
3	–$8,102	–$35,253	–$7,800	–$43,522
4	–$8,193	–$27,966	–$7,800	–$36,793
5	–$8,286	–$20,367	–$7,800	–$29,863
6	–$8,381	–$12,443	–$7,800	–$22,725
7	–$8,478	–$ 4,185	–$7,800	–$15,373
8	$4,422	$ 4,422	–$7,800	–$ 7,800
Bottom Line Result		–$52,509		–$54,754

purchasing could be expected to produce a total savings of $2,245 measured in today's dollars. This figure is found by computing the difference between the two Bottom Line Results.

The above benefit and cost analysis provides for a comprehensive summary of leasing versus purchasing, taking into account the time value of money. The analysis is so large and complex that at first it may appear nearly impossible. However, by separating the process into the stages and categories that are provided, it can be broken down into manageable parts.

Physician's Checklist

As a summary of this chapter, ask yourself the following questions. If you can answer "yes" to these questions, you have a reasonable level of understanding of leases and can make the decision of whether to buy or lease.

_____ 1. Do you understand that an operating lease if for convenient, short-term use of an asset, while a capital or finance lease usually reflects a long-term commitment similar to purchasing an asset?

_____ 2. Do you understand how depreciation is not a cash outflow but creates cash inflows by reducing income taxes?

_____ 3. Do you understand that in theory, individuals or business organizations in the highest tax brackets should purchase and those in lower tax brackets should lease?

_____ 4. Can you identify and place into a financial analysis the taxable cash flows, nontaxable cash flows, and depreciation figures for buying and leasing?

_____ 5. Can you complete the financial analysis including discounting the aggregate cash flows into a discounted Bottom Line Result?

_____ 6. Do you understand what a comparison of the Bottom Line Results means and how to make a decision of leasing versus buying?

This chapter has provided an overview of leasing and has detailed a financial analysis that can be used to make lease versus buy decisions. In fact, the financial analysis demonstrated in this chapter can be adapted to compare any two financial alternatives.

A discussion of the financial aspects of a medical practice is incomplete without consideration of the financial commitment dictated by pension plan considerations. This book concludes with a final chapter on retirement planning.

Questions and Answers

1. **What questions should I ask when I consider the purchase or lease of an asset?**

    The first question that you ask is whether the technology of the equipment is rapidly changing. If the technology changes quickly, you should consider an operating lease rather than a purchase of the asset. In addition, you should ask whether the financing alternative gives you flexibility for an upgrade or trade-in of the asset.

2. **How do I know whether leasing or buying the asset makes the best economic sense?**

    There is no easy answer to this question. In order to determine what is the appropriate approach to asset acquisition means that you have to perform a cost/benefit analysis for each of the alternatives. Thus, you need to compile the costs of each alternative and determine how each of these costs affect the cash flow in a given period. You must then discount the cash flows for the time value of money and add the net result. Only after cost/benefit analysis has been performed can you answer this vitally important question.

3. **What types of leases are there?**

    There are two types of leases: the first is an operating lease which allows you to expense the cost of leasing the equipment on a pay-as-you-go basis; however, you do not own the asset. In contrast, a financing or capital lease allows you to finance the asset as if it were a purchase. With a financing lease, you own the asset and depreciate it over its useful life.

4. **What is the impact of an operating or financing (capital) lease on my financial statements?**

    Since periodic payments are the only cash flow requirements and an operating lease charges expense when you make a payment, the cash flow impact and the impact on net income are the same. In contrast, a financing lease actually represents the purchase of the asset. With the purchase and legal title, you depreciate the asset over its useful life at an amount that most likely will differ from your cash flow requirements. Thus, the depreciation expense recorded on the Statement of Revenues and Expenses would be different from the cash outflow reported on the Statement of Cash Flows.

5. **Why does depreciation expense offer a tax "benefit" to those who own the assets?**

    Depreciation offers a tax benefit because the expense associated with owning an asset can reduce the income of the medical practice over a specified time period. Thus, taxable income is reduced, resulting in lower taxes.

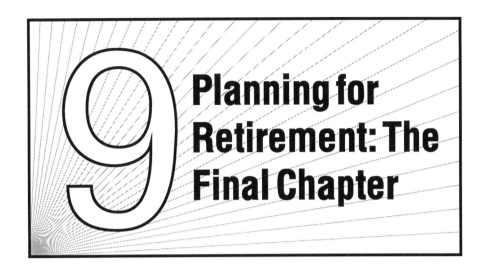

9
Planning for Retirement: The Final Chapter

Dr. Lave is feeling quite comfortable with his business affairs. Now that he has mastered the terminology and concepts of his business, he wonders if he can apply any of his newly found knowledge to his personal situation.

As he begins to think about this aspect, he thinks a good starting point is to compute his current wealth. He figures that his house and cars are worth hundreds of thousands of dollars. However, since his cars and home have significant debts attached to them, he knows that his net worth from these assets is rather small.

In reviewing his other assets, he knows that his investment account with a brokerage firm has languished for years. He also knows that his limited partnerships, purchased years ago, are now worth almost nothing. However, he has an emergency cash reserve in bank certificates of deposit worth about $20,000. Reflecting on this, he decides that it isn't much to show for over 20 years of hard work.

However, Dr. Lave remembers that he has significant retirement savings. For over 20 years, he has been placing a sizeable portion of his earnings in retirement programs earning competitive returns. He knows that his annual contributions to the various retirement plans have remained steady each year at about $20,000 per year. Even ignoring interest, he figures that his retirement funds should be worth over $400,000!

To try and verify the balance in his retirement plans, he begins to search his files for the statements that he received. He always filed them away, knowing that one day he would need them. And now is the time! He locates the statements but finds them quite confusing to read. However, armed with renewed confidence because of his new accounting and finance skills, he perseveres. His retirement funds were located in several different plans and were diversified among several well-regarded firms. After *compiling the figures, Dr. Lave discovers the powerful results of compound interest and rising stock markets: his retirement plans are currently valued at over $1,500,000!*

Dr. Lave's situation is not all that unusual. Many Americans find that retirement plans are the single most important part of their wealth accumulation and financial security. If more Americans truly understood the advantages of accumulating wealth in retirement plans, they would be utilized even more.

The most important benefit from retirement investing is the enormity of its tax advantages. Many people think that retirement plans merely allow investors to earn investment returns and save taxes. However, retirement investing can actually be tax subsidized! The amazing tax benefits of retirement investing will be demonstrated later in the chapter. For now, let's overview some of the other aspects.

Specifically, this chapter will address the following questions:

- What are the types of retirement plans?
- What is a defined contribution and defined benefit plan?
- What are the tax benefits from pension investing?
- How much retirement savings is enough?
- What investment management practices should be followed?

What Are the Types of Retirement Plans?

The "Big Picture," Legally Speaking

Currently, there is no law to prevent a person from saving for retirement using funds "outside" of retirement plans, such as buying and holding gold coins in their basement. (Although this was against the law in America earlier this century.) Thus, in a technical sense, a person can be said to be investing for retirement whenever they invest in a house or other asset whose usefulness might extend into their retirement years.

However, for most people it is important to enjoy the tax advantages offered by "formal" retirement plans. In other words, when we refer to retirement investing we are referring to retirement plans approved by the Internal Revenue Service (IRS) for tax benefits ("qualified plans"). The legal and accounting complexities of retirement plans can be viewed as the bureaucratic price that must be paid if you want to enjoy the tax benefits of traditional retirement plans.

In 1974, Congress enacted ERISA (the Employee Retirement Income Security Act) to prevent misuses. Further, the benefits of some plans are insured by a government agency (the Pension Benefit Guaranty Corporation or PBGC). This involvement of the government in general, and the IRS in particular, is why the remaining material in this section is complex.

First, there are numerous types of plans. Which type of retirement plan should you use?

There is an "alphabet soup" of alternative retirement plans available. Those applicable to physicians or medical practices are:

- Simplified Employee Pension (SEP)—A retirement plan which allows you to make contributions for both you and your employees based on compensation.
- Keogh—A retirement plan for a sole proprietor or partnership for the exclusive benefit of the employees. Individual partners cannot set up a Keogh.
- 401(k)—A retirement plan in the form of a savings plan applicable to all organizations.
- Individual Retirement Arrangements (IRA)—A retirement plan option for any individual who receives compensation during a year.

It is important to note that each of these plans has various operating requirements and restrictions as well as different tax effects. Extensive information has been written on these plans and their advantages and disadvantages are summarized in Figure 9-1.

Figure 9-1 is indicative of the legal and accounting complexities of retirement plans. Deciding which plan is right for you and your medical practice depends upon your circumstances and current regulations. Unfortunately, new plans are created and the rules governing the old plans can change rapidly. Thus, it is inappropriate for this book to offer specific prescriptions.

Which type of plan to use must ultimately be decided with assistance from a professional who specializes in the area and is current with the legal and tax implications. In order to assist you in approaching a professional, we will overview the information available at the time of this writing.

A useful starting point for discussion with your professional is to investigate defined contribution plans (to be discussed later) that offer the least legal and accounting complexity, while permitting the desired level of contributions. For a small practice with limited contributions, a SEP might be best due to its potentially lower costs. For larger plans, and/or for practices seeking large contribution limits, a Keogh might be best. There are several types of Keoghs, including profit sharing, money purchase, and defined benefit.

FIGURE 9-1
VARIOUS RETIREMENT PLANS

TYPE	ADVANTAGES/DISADVANTAGES
Simplified Employee Pension (SEP)	Very simple, moderate maximum contribution limits
Keogh	Moderately simple, many types, generous maximum contribution limits
401(k)	Flexible, moderate maximum contribution levels
Individual Retirement Account (IRA)	Simple, but tight restrictions on tax deductibility of contributions

Nontax Benefits of Pension Programs

There are reasons other than taxes for establishing pension programs. Obviously, retirement programs can guide you and your employees towards planning for the future.

Retirement programs can also provide financial protection against financial disasters such as lawsuits, poor financial planning, and bad economic times. Although the laws vary from state to state, most retirement plans are protected from creditors and claimants in bankruptcy. Thus, a person can pass through bankruptcy, discharging debts and legal claims while retaining most or all of their retirement money.

In plain English, depending upon your state, retirement plans can offer a tremendous vehicle for wealth accumulation that might be protected from some financial disasters such as lawsuits and business failures.

General Considerations and ERISA

Funds placed into retirement plans can be restricted or penalized substantially if withdrawn earlier than retirement age (now typically age 59½). These laws can change and can even be applied to funds that were placed into the plan before any restrictions had been imposed.

ERISA and other legislation affect relative treatment of employees and what happens when an employee leaves the firm or the firm ceases to exist. A competent professional should be consulted on a regular basis.

What Is a Defined Contribution and Defined Benefit Plan?

One of the most important distinctions between retirement plans is the difference between defined benefit and defined contribution plans. Most modern retirement plans are defined contribution plans.

Defined Benefit Plans

Defined benefit plans are often viewed as "old-fashioned" pensions whereby an employee receives a retirement income based upon years of service. For example, an employee might receive a fixed pension equal to 2 percent of his or her final salary for each year of service. Thus an employee with 30 years of service might retire at 60 percent pay.

The key to this type of plan is that the employee's pension (i.e., the benefit) is defined or fixed on a basis such as years of service and final salary.

By guaranteeing a particular benefit, an enormous risk is taken with regard to the investment returns that need to be earned on the pension funds throughout the employee's career. This risk can be borne by the employer, or passed on to a financial firm, but ultimately someone must pay for this risk.

Imagine trying to figure out how much money should be set aside today, on behalf of a 25-year-old, to meet a benefit that might not even begin to be paid out for 40 years? What happens if investment returns fall and the pension funds set aside during the employee's career fail to provide for the promised benefit?

However, the employer is required to meet the benefit regardless of investment performance. If the employer is unable to meet the obligation, the government may step in or the employee may be out of luck.

Other problems with defined benefit plans include the impact of employees switching jobs and the likelihood that the pension benefit will be relatively fixed during retirement and therefore open to the risk of high inflation rates.

Defined Contribution Plans

The other major category of retirement plans is defined contribution plans. These plans are like individual savings accounts. The amount of money placed into the plans each year is determined for each employee—hence the name defined contribution. However, the amount of pension income, or benefit, that these contributions eventually produce depends upon the size of the contributions, market conditions, investment choices, and so forth. Defined contribution plans are simpler, less risky, and increasingly popular.

What Are the Tax Benefits from Pension Investing?

The power of the tax benefits of retirement programs is amazing—so amazing that they often must be seen to be believed. Years ago, one of this book's authors had recently completed a graduate business education and, like most professors, was contributing the standard, minimum dollars towards a pension plan. One day, he was asked to correct a large, but difficult to find, "error" in a computer program that illustrated tax benefits of pension saving. The computer program was saying that a person can earn enormous after-tax returns from pension investing even when the assets inside the pension plan are earning poor returns before tax.

After a great deal of analysis, it was revealed that the computer program was indeed correct. The program demonstrated such amazing tax benefits that the author immediately increased pension funding from the minimum to the maximum. We hope that you, too, will understand these benefits and do likewise. This section will demonstrate those tax advantages with a numerical example.

Tax Deferral

To begin, retirement plan investing gives you a tax deferral (i.e., the delay of the payment of taxes from one year to a later year). When $100 is placed into a pension plan and begins to earn interest, the interest is not taxed until the money is withdrawn from the plan. However, when $100 is invested into a normal account, the interest will be taxed each year and will not be able to fully compound. Therefore, the full interest amount earns "interest on interest" without taxation (until withdrawal).

This deferral of taxation until withdrawal may seem like a small issue since in many cases the income taxes must be paid either way. In fact, some rather financially conservative people actually have an initial reaction of wanting to pay the taxes "now" to "get them out of the way."

However, since retirement plans are generally long term, the ability to defer taxes and earn interest on the full amount, can be significant. The power of this tax deferral benefit is shown in Figure 9-2.

Figure 9-2 demonstrates after-tax accumulation, with and without tax deferral, for periods of 1, 10 and 40 years. We use a tax rate of 35 percent to represent a typical combination of Federal, state, and local income tax rates for people with moderately high incomes.

Throughout this chapter we focus on individual income taxes. However, if your form of business organization (see Chapter 2) is taxed on income, then additional potential tax savings may be available. Further, retirement savings can offer protection from other types of taxes such as social security contributions.

Figure 9-2 shows that over a period of one year there is no advantage to tax deferral since income taxes are paid immediately either way. Note that both without deferral and with deferral, the after tax accumulation value is $1,065. Over a period of 10 years the tax deferral begins to become significant.

FIGURE 9-2
THE POWER OF TAX DEFERRAL ONLY
Pension Benefit from a One-Time $1,000 Contribution
10 Percent Investment Returns and a 35 Percent Tax Rate

	Number of Years		
	1	10	40
WITHOUT DEFERRAL:			
Contribution	$1,000	$1,000	$ 1,000
Annual Growth Rate*	6.5%	6.5%	6.5%
Contribution plus Interest	$1,065	$1,877	$12,416
Less Taxes on Withdrawal	$0	$0	$0
After Tax Value	$1,065	$1,877	$12,416
WITH DEFERRAL:			
Contribution	$1,000	$1,000	$ 1,000
Annual Growth Rate	10%	10%	10%
Contribution plus Interest	$1,100	$2,594	$45,259
Less Taxes on Withdrawal	$35	$558	$15,491
After Tax Value	$1,065	$2,036	$29,769
DOLLAR ADVANTAGE OF DEFERRAL	$0	$159	$17,353

* Note: If 35 percent income taxes are paid each year out of the investment income of 10 percent per year, there will be an after tax growth rate of 6.5 percent.

However, note that with a time horizon of 40 years and an interest rate of 10 percent, the advantage of tax deferral explodes. Without deferral the account grows to $12,416 after taxes. However, with tax deferral the account grows to $29,769—a $17,353 improvement! The tax deferred plan generates more than twice the after tax retirement income—it just doesn't seem possible!

As we look into a future of later retirement ages and longer life spans, an employee who starts contributing at age 25 probably will retire at age 65 or later. At that point, they have a reasonable likelihood of either living to age 90 or having a spouse live that long. Thus, some money might be in the retirement plan for 65 years!

It is currently possible to enjoy the tax benefits of tax deferral without contributing to retirement plans, for example, through life insurance plans. However, tax deferral is just the start of the tax benefit to retirement investing.

Tax Deductibility

The biggest tax advantage to retirement investing is your ability to deduct current contributions from current taxable income.

For example, suppose that an investor works for numerous years, has a pension plan, and then retires and withdraws from the pension plan while being taxed at the same tax rate that he or she contributed at while working. In this case, the retirement plan produces such enormous tax benefits that it effectively offers tax-free investing.

This equivalent of tax-free investing can be achieved without being forced to accept the low yields that ordinary tax-free investments, such as municipal bonds, offer.

It may be difficult to believe that retirement investing is free of taxes if you have the same tax rate before and after retirement, but it's true. The reason is that tax deduction, combined with tax deferral, is equivalent to tax free.

For example, consider an investor who is working and who contributes $1,000 into a retirement plan. Because the contribution is tax deductible he or she receives an immediate reduction in taxes of $350 if he or she is in a 35 percent tax bracket. Thus, the investor has really only given up $650 but has $1,000 inside the retirement plan.

First, let's look at *not* using a retirement plan. If the investor didn't put the $1,000 in the retirement plan, then he or she would have to use $350 to pay taxes. If he or she put the remaining $650 in a 10 percent tax-free account for 40 years, the money would grow to $29,419.

Now, let's return to what happens if the investor uses a retirement plan. Assume that he or she places the full $1,000 in a plan paying 10 percent. Forty years later the investor withdraws the money and its interest and pays 35 percent taxes on both the original contribution and its growth. Notice that the tax savings increase the funds available for the original contribution while the taxes on the withdrawal decrease the funds available at retirement. We will show that these two effects can offset each other leaving the plan free of taxation.

For example, if he or she had invested at 10 percent for 40 years, the investor's $1,000 retirement plan would have increased in value to $45,259. After withdrawing the money and paying 35 percent taxes on the full withdrawal ($15,841 = $45,259 * 35%) the investor would be left with $29,419. But $29,419 of after-tax retirement spending money is exactly the same figure that we obtained using no taxes. It reflects exactly a 10 percent annual increase relative to his or her actual $650 of after-tax spending money which he or she sacrificed during his or her working years. Thus, on an after-tax basis the investor earned 10 percent!

The point of the above example is that retirement plans are far more powerful than "tax-advantaged." They do not simply lower taxes on investment income; they can eliminate them. Remember, this plan allowed the investor to obtain tax-free investment returns. This occurred without having to accept the lower yields that an investor would normally have if he or she invested in ordinary tax-free alternatives such as municipal bonds.

To summarize, elimination of income taxes on investment income occurs when individuals contribute to retirement plans, enjoy tax deductibility and tax deferral, and then withdraw the funds at retirement while in the same tax bracket (i.e., paying taxes at the same tax rate).

Tax Subsidized Investing

The previous subsection demonstrated that retirement plans not only reduce investment income taxes, they can eliminate them. This subsection will go one step further and show how retirement plans can be *tax subsidized*.

If the tax bracket paid during the retirement (withdrawal) period is lower than during the working years—as it usually is—then retirement plans are better than tax-free; they are actually tax subsidized investments!

In other words, if your tax bracket at retirement is *lower* than during contribution, then retirement plans offer higher after-tax returns than the before-tax yield of the underlying investments. You can invest in CDs yielding 8 percent and effectively earn better than 8 percent when taxes are included in the analysis. This is tax subsidized investing!

Figure 9-3 illustrates this point by showing the after-tax rates of returns earned by an investor who contributes to a plan when his or her tax rate is 35 percent, and withdraws from the plan when the tax rate has fallen to 15 percent (retirement).

Figure 9-3 indicates that if you invest in a pension plan that earns 10 percent for five years, you will receive a return of 16.1 percent after taxes if you contribute while your combined tax ratios are 35 percent and withdraw when your combined rates are 15 percent!

Figure 9-3 is so surprising that it deserves close inspection. The example assumes that the investor's retirement contributions were tax deductible during his or her working years at a tax rate of 35 percent. When the investor retired, his or her tax rate dropped to 15 percent.

Recall that a $1,000 retirement contribution really only costs the worker $650 because it saves him or her $350 in the current year's income taxes. However, the full $1,000 enters the retirement plan and earns interest. When withdrawn, it is all taxed at a potentially lower rate (e.g., 15 percent).

Let's pursue the example of this $1,000 retirement contribution (that really only costs the investor $650) for someone retiring in one year and investing in a one year

FIGURE 9-3
AFTER-TAX RATE OF RETURN FOR INVESTOR WITH
FALLING TAX RATES

Number of Years between Contribution and Withdrawal	After-Tax Rate of Return with a Pretax Rate of Return of 10%
1	43.8%
5	16.1%
10	13.0%
20	11.5%

CD earning 10 percent. When the worker retires in one year and earns 10 percent interest, his or her retirement plan will have grown to $1,100. The withdrawal of this $1,100 will create increased taxes of 15 percent of the withdrawal or $165—leaving the retiree with $935 to spend.

The $935 that can be withdrawn (after tax) only cost the retiree $650 in after-tax cash flow. Since the transaction lasted only one year it is therefore a return of 43.8 percent: [($935–$650)/$650]. Thus, 43.8 percent is shown in the first row of the entries in Figure 9-3.

A typical investor can earn 11–44 percent after taxes by buying bonds in a retirement plan that yield only 10 percent! The yield is effectively being subsidized by reduced and deferred income taxes on wages.

The ability to earn a greater after-tax return than the underlying investments are yielding results primarily from the tax windfall of deducting money now at a tax rate of 35 percent and declaring it much later at a tax rate of only 15 percent. This can be viewed as a long-term, interest-free loan which only needs to be partially repaid.

Is it reasonable to expect that tax rates will be lower in the retirement years than in the working years? Well, it is impossible to predict long-range income tax rates, but there are three things working in the favor of the retirement investor. First, most people retire at a lower income level than they earned during their working years. Thus, some investors will find their tax brackets lower due to lower income. Second, some people move to states, such as Florida, that have lower state income tax rates or no state income tax. Third, careful estate planning can often allow retirees to pass their retirement savings to beneficiaries through their estate and avoid income taxes completely.

Summary of Tax Benefits

When considering retirement planning, one of the most important aspects is to fully comprehend the extent of the tax benefits available through retirement investing. For most investors in high tax brackets, full funding of retirement plans should be the highest investment priority.

An investor can use retirement plans to earn after-tax rate of returns which significantly exceed the before-tax rate of return of fully taxable investments. Wise people agree: the surest path to significant wealth is gradual accumulation. Retirement investing is the ideal vehicle for that objective.

How Much Retirement Savings Is Enough?

One of the problems with defined contribution retirement plans is that people have difficulty assessing how much money is needed in order to receive a given benefit. This section will address this issue in two ways.

First, we will evaluate what percentage of a person's income should be contributed throughout the worker's career. Second, we will consider the dollar amount that should be accumulated at each point in the career.

What Percentage of a Salary Should Be Contributed to a Retirement Plan?

Many variables affect the determination of an appropriate percentage of salary that should be placed into a retirement plan. The worst problem is that the future returns on the investments are unknown relative to the inflation rate. Nevertheless, we must do the best we can. Figure 9-4 suggests reasonable estimates of appropriate contribution rates for various situations.

FIGURE 9-4
CONTRIBUTION RATES TO RETIRE AT 60% OF INCOME

		Annual Average Returns Net of Inflation		
Contributing Years	Retirement Years	1% (Poor)	4% (Average)	7% (Good)
15	10	35.30%	24.30%	16.77%
15	20	67.26%	40.72%	25.30%
15	30	96.20%	51.81%	29.63%
25	10	20.12%	11.69%	6.66%
25	20	38.34%	19.58%	10.05%
25	30	54.83%	24.91%	11.77%
35	10	13.64%	6.61%	3.05%
35	20	25.99%	11.07%	4.60%
35	30	37.17%	14.09%	5.39%

The numbers should not be taken too literally. The years of contribution have been broken into three categories: 15 years, 25 years, and 35 years, representing an approximation of how many years a worker plans to realistically contribute to a defined contribution program.

The number of retirement years has also been divided into three categories in order to approximate reasonable forecasts of retirement (or at least healthy retirement), given various retirement ages and health expectations.

The critical forecast is the rate of return that the retirement plan will offer relative to inflation. We have considered three levels: 1 percent, 4 percent, and 7 percent, corresponding to poor, average, and good returns.

For example, the selection of 1 percent would be a highly conservative forecast of future investment returns relative to inflation. The use of this figure indicates that the investor anticipates receiving investment returns that average only 1 percent greater than the inflation rate. This might occur if the investor selects extremely conservative investment choices such as money market mutual funds or if the investor selects higher risk choices and the economy (or his or her particular investments) perform poorly for an extended period of time.

The middle level of 4 percent is intended as a long-range forecast of after inflation return for a typical investor with investments split between stocks and bonds. This assumes that an extended time line with several business cycles will be spanned and that the investor becomes more conservative in investing near and during the retirement years.

Finally, the highest level of 7% is an optimistic but highly possible after inflation return for an aggressive investor who retains high percentages of stocks, even during retirement, and who benefits from a healthy economy.

We recommend that you select the level or levels that most closely match your investment strategy. Then compare your numbers with other levels to get a "feel" for what would happen if investment returns turn out better or worse than expected.

For example, a worker who starts contributing to retirement plans while relatively young and who plans to retire at a normal retirement age might find the second to last line of the table useful. It would indicate the need to put between 4.6 and 26 percent of current income into retirement plans.

The top two-thirds of Figure 9-4 demonstrate the importance of planning for retirement at an early age. The differences between the columns highlight the significance of earning a decent rate of return relative to inflation. The prescription for retirement can be summarized: start early, invest wisely, or die quickly!

It is important to note that Figure 9-4 indicates the contributions necessary to fund a retirement at 60 percent of the average income (don't worry about inflation) that was received during the years of contribution. Many people use this figure as a reasonable estimate of how much money is needed for a pleasant retirement above and beyond social security and perhaps having already put the kids through college, paid off the mortgage, saved for retirement, and so forth.

The figures in the table can be adjusted upward or downward to reflect different percentages. For example, if you desire to retire at the same income and do not anticipate social security, multiply each figure by 1.67 since 1.67 times 60 percent equals 100 percent (rounded).

How Much Money Should I Currently Have Accumulated for Retirement?

Another important issue is how much retirement savings a person should have accumulated at various points in time. As we discussed in the previous subsection, this answer depends upon numerous variables. We can only do our best with limited ability to forecast how long we will live, or how great investment returns will be relative to inflation.

We constructed three figures that cover a variety of rates of investment returns and retirement time spans. The three tables correspond to three retirement assumptions: retirement for 10 years at age 65, retirement for 20 years at age 60, and retirement for 30 years at age 58.

The first, Figure 9-5, should be viewed as the funds that should be accumulated for a modest retirement, such as a 10-year retirement at age 65 with $50,000 per year, or other combinations involving longer retirements with lower income.

The second, Figure 9-6, corresponds to a more normal retirement of 20 years, beginning at age 60. The last of the three, Figure 9-7, corresponds to a luxurious retirement of 30 years, beginning at age 58.

We assumed the same rates of return used in the previous subsection (1 percent, 4 percent, and 7 percent net of inflation), which represent conservative, moderate, and aggressive return expectations. Each figure incorporates the point at which the retirement contributions began.

Each figure lists the amount of accumulation that would be needed to produce $50,000 of retirement income in today's dollars and continuing on an inflation adjusted basis. In other words, think about today's dollars and totally ignore inflation (the higher prices when you retire). If you plan on more or less than $50,000 of retirement income (above and beyond social security and any defined benefit plans) then simply adjust the figures accordingly. A $75,000 income is found by multiplying the figures by 1.5 and a $25,000 income is found by multiplying the figures by 0.5.

There are several ways of using the figures. First, you may wish to determine where you should be in terms of accumulated retirement savings. This should be done with consideration of the age that you began contributing, your current age, your forecast of investment returns, and your retirement plans.

Alternatively, you may experiment with the retirement ages and investment returns that relate to the actual level of accumulated retirement savings. This might guide the reader in investment decisions and retirement plans.

For example, assume you are a 40-year-old and wish to retire with $25,000 income (measured in today's spending power) above and beyond social security. You have been saving since you were 25 years old and you have accumulated $150,000 in retirement savings. How are you doing?

First, since you only forecast a need for $25,000 per year retirement income and since the table is based upon $50,000, we can mentally divide all of the entries in Figures

FIGURE 9-5
MODEST RETIREMENT NEEDS
Accumulation Amounts to Retire at $50,000 Income
with Short Retirement (10 Years) at Age 65

Began at Age	Current Age	Annual Average Returns Net of Inflation		
		1% (Poor)	4% (Average)	7% (Good)
25	30	$49,414	$23,115	$10,116
25	35	$101,348	$51,239	$24,305
25	40	$155,932	$85,456	$44,205
25	45	$213,299	$127,085	$72,115
25	50	$273,594	$177,734	$111,262
25	55	$336,963	$239,356	$166,166
25	60	$403,566	$314,329	$243,173
25	65	$473,565	$405,545	$351,179
30	35	$57,985	$29,823	$14,609
30	40	$118,927	$66,108	$35,100
30	45	$182,978	$110,254	$63,838
30	50	$250,297	$163,964	$104,146
30	55	$321,049	$229,311	$160,679
30	60	$395,411	$308,816	$239,970
30	65	$473,565	$405,545	$351,179
35	40	$69,446	$39,165	$21,380
35	45	$142,434	$86,815	$51,366
35	50	$219,145	$144,789	$93,423
35	55	$299,769	$215,322	$153,410
35	60	$384,506	$301,138	$235,142
35	65	$473,565	$405,545	$351,179
40	45	$85,531	$52,744	$31,930
40	50	$175,424	$116,915	$76,713
40	55	$269,903	$194,988	$139,524
40	60	$369,202	$289,977	$227,620
40	65	$473,565	$405,545	$351,179
45	50	$109,708	$73,764	$49,262
45	55	$225,012	$163,510	$118,356
45	60	$346,198	$272,699	$215,262
45	65	$473,565	$405,545	$351,179
50	55	$150,070	$109,699	$80,367
50	60	$307,795	$243,164	$193,085
50	65	$473,565	$405,545	$351,179
55	60	$230,894	$182,954	$146,169
55	65	$473,565	$405,545	$351,179
60	65	$473,565	$405,545	$351,179

FIGURE 9-6
NORMAL RETIREMENT NEEDS
Accumulation Amounts to Retire at $50,000 Income
with Moderate Retirement (20 Years) at Age 60

Began at Age	Current Age	1% (Poor)	4% (Average)	7% (Good)
			Annual Average Returns Net of Inflation	
25	30	$110,477	$49,971	$22,036
25	35	$226,590	$110,768	$52,942
25	40	$348,626	$184,738	$96,290
25	45	$476,887	$274,733	$157,088
25	50	$611,691	$384,226	$242,360
25	55	$753,371	$571,440	$361,958
25	60	$902,278	$679,516	$529,701
30	35	$132,314	$65,623	$32,248
30	40	$271,377	$145,464	$77,477
30	45	$417,534	$242,603	$140,914
30	50	$571,146	$360,787	$229,887
30	55	$732,594	$504,575	$354,677
30	60	$902,278	$679,516	$529,701
35	40	$162,960	$88,376	$48,162
35	45	$334,233	$195,898	$115,711
35	50	$514,243	$326,715	$210,452
35	55	$703,435	$485,875	$343,331
35	60	$902,278	$679,516	$529,701
40	45	$209,025	$123,597	$74,305
40	50	$428,712	$273,972	$178,522
40	55	$659,606	$456,925	$324,691
40	60	$902,278	$679,516	$529,701
45	50	$285,926	$183,807	$121,221
45	55	$586,437	$407,437	$291,240
45	60	$902,278	$679,516	$529,701
50	55	$439,919	$306,551	$220,474
50	60	$902,278	$679,516	$529,701
55	60	$902,278	$679,516	$529,701

FIGURE 9-7
LUXURIOUS RETIREMENT NEEDS
Accumulation Amounts to Retire at $50,000 Income
with Long Retirement (30 Years) at Age 58

Began at Age	Current Age	Annual Average Returns Net of Inflation		
		1% (Poor)	4% (Average)	7% (Good)
25	30	$169,345	$70,729	$30,000
25	35	$347,328	$156,783	$72,078
25	40	$534,390	$261,479	$131,093
25	45	$730,994	$388,859	$213,865
25	50	$937,627	$543,836	$329,958
25	55	$1,154,800	$732,389	$492,783
25	58	$1,290,385	$064,602	$620,452
30	35	$204,869	$93,720	$44,215
30	40	$420,189	$207,745	$106,229
30	45	$646,492	$346,473	$193,207
30	50	$884,339	$515,258	$315,198
30	55	$1,134,318	$720,610	$486,296
30	58	$1,290,385	$864,602	$620,452
35	40	$255,957	$127,887	$66,772
35	45	$524,970	$283,482	$160,424
35	50	$807,706	$472,786	$291,775
35	55	$1,104,863	$703,104	$476,003
35	58	$1,290,385	$864,602	$620,452
40	45	$334,577	$182,604	$104,946
40	50	$688,272	$404,770	$252,138
40	55	$1,058,958	$675,069	$458,582
40	58	$1,290,385	$864,602	$620,452
45	50	$476,653	$281,651	$177,157
45	55	$977,621	$624,322	$425,629
45	58	$1,290,385	$864,602	$620,452
50	55	$794,415	$508,232	$347,771
50	58	$1,290,385	$864,602	$620,452
55	58	$1,290,385	$864,602	$620,452

9-5 through 9-7 by two to reflect your need for only half of the income that the figures were based upon.

Next, given your current age of 40 and your history of having started your retirement savings at age 25, you locate the third row of each table. You note that your actual retirement savings ($150,000) greatly exceeds all of the entries in Figure 9-5 (remembering to divide each entry in half). Thus, you are financially well ahead of a plan for a short, modest retirement, even if investment returns are poor.

Next, inspect Figure 9-6 for the purpose of comparing your retirement savings to a more normal retirement. Halving each entry, you find that your $150,000 savings exceeds the target for 4 percent returns and falls a little short of the target for 1 percent returns. Thus, you are financially ahead of a plan for a normal retirement if returns are normal or even significantly below normal. However, rather poor investment returns could leave you a little short of your goal.

Finally, inspect Figure 9-7 for the purpose of comparing your retirement savings relative to a luxurious or early retirement. Halving each entry, you find that you are on target given normal returns, but would fall far short of a luxurious or early retirement if returns fall significantly below normal.

Notice that this analysis not only can guide you to understanding where you currently stand in your financial retirement plan, but it can also be used to provide guidance with regard to the level of aggressiveness with which to invest. An aggressive, higher risk investment strategy increases the probability of higher returns and lower returns.

The tables allow you to compare the retirement prospects for alternative investment strategies. By becoming more aggressive (i.e., investing substantially in long-term common stock holdings) an investor will typically significantly increase the average return. However, an aggressive strategy can also increase the probability of poor returns.

This leads us to one of the most important and misunderstood aspects of retirement: investment management.

What Investment Management Practices Should Be Followed?

Health care professionals often find themselves in a position of making investment decisions on their own behalf and often on behalf of their employees. This section provides an overview of the major decisions.

Before exploring the details of retirement investment management, it is useful to consider the "big picture" or the investment philosophy.

Competent long-run investment management is the result of a consistent, thoughtful, traditional and informed decision-making process rather than new or get rich quick schemes.

As a medical professional, you probably suggest that patients seeking physical health follow established and proven methods of promoting long-term health rather than jumping into fads that promise miraculous healings. The same concepts apply to financial health.

Common sense should be applied not only to the methods used, but also the selection of the people that will be entrusted with investment management. Many of the same concepts that you as a medical professional would suggest with regard to how to select competent professional medical care can be used to select competent investment management professionals. However, one very important result of common sense deserves emphasis: if a person truly has a method of producing vastly superior investment results, they will keep it a secret and make a fortune for themselves rather than attempt to find other people's money to invest.

The legal system generally does not protect people from investment mistakes. Business owners can not only harm themselves financially, but they might have a fiduciary responsibility to their employees with regard to pension investment management. Accordingly, we urge you to adopt proven and prudent investment strategies and to apply them with a long-term focus.

The Fixed Income/Equity Mix

The most important investment decision in managing retirement investments is the allocation of the funds between fixed incomes and equities.

Fixed income alternatives include those securities that offer relatively fixed or predetermined rates of return. Examples include bank certificates of deposit, money market mutual funds, bonds, bond funds, and annuities.

Equities are essentially common stock and investment vehicles linked to common stocks such as equity mutual funds. Equity securities are a claim to ownership and therefore they offer future returns that are strongly based upon the future performance of the underlying companies and the markets.

Equity securities are typically viewed as the high risk alternative and most fixed income alternatives are typically viewed as relatively far less risky. However, over the long run, most equity alternatives provide better inflation protection than many fixed income alternatives.

Many experts believe that the long-run superiority of equity performance in the past supports the idea that a retirement investor should put the highest possible percentage of their funds into equity that can be tolerated in a risk sense.

Some people approach the mix between equities and fixed income securities as a high stakes and complicated guessing game in which various opinions are collected and analyzed regarding forecasts of future performance.

However, retirement money should be invested using solid investment practices rather than subjected to speculation based upon opinions of the future. A mix should be adopted based upon a thoughtful analysis of risk and that mix should only be adjusted as personal circumstances change, usually slowly.

We suggest that the percentage of the retirement funds placed in equity investments be linked to the time horizon of the beneficiary, the beneficiary's financial situation, and the beneficiary's attitude towards risk.

The investor's investment horizon is the number of years that they anticipate before the money will be used. Note that retirement money is used throughout retirement and not just at the point of retirement. Thus, some of the money placed in a retirement program by a 25-year-old may not be withdrawn until 60 years later.

Figure 9-8 illustrates the concept that the percentage of retirement funds exposed to the higher risk of equity should decline as the beneficiary approaches retirement and perhaps even decline throughout the retirement years. Thus, many people may contribute almost entirely to equity alternatives in the earliest years of their career and then move almost completely to fixed income securities in their retirement years.

However, the number of years before the money will probably be needed is only one determinant. A person in tight financial circumstances unable to experience large losses or a person with a low emotional tolerance for risk would typically prefer a lower percentage of equities than a person with a more secure financial situation and with a more aggressive attitude.

The decision is extremely critical and conventional wisdom should be considered. The classic retirement fund mix appears to have shifted from 50 percent/50 percent to 60 percent/40 percent in favor of equities. However, as discussed above, actual allocations should be based upon time horizon and attitudes towards risk.

In Figure 9-8, the concept of individuals with different tolerance of risk is expressed by showing a higher risk tolerance with x's and a lower risk tolerance with y's. Notice, the mix does not change based upon beliefs that the market is "too high," has "bottomed out," and so forth. Anybody who can consistently forecast the future direction of the stock market can earn a fortune starting with a small amount of money using options and futures. If these people succeed, they keep their mouths shut. If they fail, they look for fools with money to invest in their next scheme.

FIGURE 9-8
INVESTMENT MIX AS DETERMINED BY THE NUMBER OF YEARS UNTIL THE MONEY IS NEEDED (INVESTMENT HORIZON)

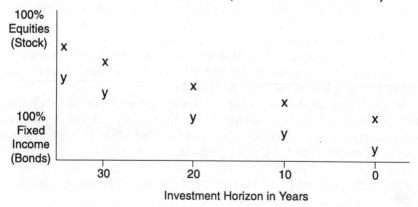

Mutual Funds

One of the most popular investment vehicles is the mutual fund. A mutual fund is simply a corporation that pools funds from many investors and manages the funds with specific investment objectives. Some mutual funds, such as money market mutual funds, are extremely low risk. Mutual funds consisting of equities, fixed income securities, or a mix are very popular.

The investor in a mutual fund receives whatever rate of return that the investments within the fund produce (minus fund expenses, management fees, and perhaps sales charges).

Mutual funds are extremely useful—especially for small to moderate-sized retirement plans such as less than $10 million.

It is obvious that mutual funds should be selected with investment objectives that match the desires of the investor. Thus, it would be typical for each employee to have a choice of funds (i.e., stock, bonds, balanced, money markets, international) between which to allocate funds. Diversification, the process of spreading investment funds in many varied securities, is essential within each fund.

However, it is also important to select funds based upon other considerations. When a sales representative is used to select a fund, there will be sales charges deducted from investment returns when the funds are contributed (a front-end load), while the funds are being managed (a 12b-1 fee), or when withdrawn (a deferred sales charge).

The sales charges can be avoided by selecting a "no-load" mutual fund without the help of a salesperson (although technically speaking some "no load" mutual funds have up to 0.25 percent per year sales charges distributed). Obviously, if the mutual fund selection decision can be made without a salesperson or a 12b-1 fee, money can be saved.

Another important aspect of mutual funds selection is expense and management fee minimization. Remember, fees and expenses are deducted before returns are credited. The fees and expenses from past years can be found in the mutual fund's financial reports, reference materials on the mutual fund industry, and articles from periodicals.

The worst reason to select a mutual fund is superior recent return performance. The best performing funds of the short-term past are less likely to be the best performing funds of the future. Fools switch from fund to fund searching for a winner.

With thousands of mutual funds available, the decision can be difficult. There is a clear strategy for long-run success. We suggest that you select funds with appropriate investment objectives from huge nationally known families of no-load mutual funds with a tradition of low management fees and expenses.

Insurance Annuities and Other Financial Institutions

Another investment alternative is to invest through insurance companies and other financial institutions offering annuities and investment contracts. These programs are especially useful for smaller plans and for participants desiring fixed income alternatives.

Insurance companies serve as a financial intermediary between the investor and the securities. They can offer useful services such as payouts that are based upon life expectancies and that continue for actual lifetimes.

Well-capitalized insurance companies can also add safety. However, some insurance companies are not very safe and can ultimately be located in offshore "free banking" havens. Major insurance companies are closely regulated and are rated for safety in publications such as Best's. It is essential to deal only with the highest rated firms (verify them yourself).

Finally, remember that insurance companies offer their services for a fee that ultimately comes out of the investment returns. There are no free lunches!

Stock Brokers and Investment Managers

A final category of investment vehicles considered includes stock brokers and investment managers or advisors. Stock brokers tend to be used by smaller investors and investment advisors by larger investors.

It is possible to have your retirement funds managed by a stock broker from a stock brokerage firm ranging from the huge nationally known firms to the small locally operated firms. Stock brokers are typically compensated by commission on each trade executed for the account.

The commission can be an explicit commission shown on each trade ticket or an implicit commission built into the price of the security on a trade in which the broker serves as a "principal." Generally, the stock broker earns a larger commission whenever riskier types of securities are being traded.

For example, certificates of deposit and nationally known stocks typically produce very small commissions and are typically traded infrequently. Limited partnerships, options, some mutual funds, and small growth stocks can offer huge commissions (and huge risks) and are sometimes rapidly traded.

Great caution should be exercised in utilizing a commission-based investment professional. Such relationships run the risk of excessive trading and trading in more speculative securities. Derivatives and limited partnerships are examples of investment alternatives through which billions of dollars, including many retirement dollars, have been squandered.

Customers are almost always required to sign arbitration agreements prior to investing and many experts believe that these arbitration clauses greatly limit the legal recourse to investment problems. The expression "buyer beware" often applies.

Investment management firms or investment advisors can be arranged for a relatively fixed fee such as a percentage of assets under management. The fee can range from a high of 1–2 percent per year for small, aggressively managed relationships to 0.50 percent or less per year for larger, more conservatively managed relationships.

Most investment advisors will not consider taking on a small client, such as less than $100,000, and many have higher minimums such as $250,000, $500,000, $1,000,000, or more.

Investment managers serve as an advisor between the client and the brokerage community. Most investment advisors also have implicit or explicit arrangements through which they receive some (usually minor) economic benefit from trading customer funds through arrangements with brokerage firms. Thus, most arrangements offer some degree of a conflict of interest and unnecessary or inappropriate trading is possible. Even funds managed by investment management firms need to be monitored closely for appropriateness of risk, performance, and appropriateness of trading.

Conclusion

There is no "one size fits all" prescription for investment management of retirement funds. Perhaps the surest advice would be the use of huge nationally known families of no-load mutual funds with a history of low management fees and expenses. Funds should be selected that offer the broadest possible portfolios and investment objectives in line with your retirement plans. These investment objectives should seek long-term accumulation of funds through diversified and established means.

Physician's Checklist

As a summary of this chapter, ask yourself the following questions with respect to your pension plan and the retirement plan of your medical practice. If you can answer "yes" to these questions, then you should have a solid foundation of the major principles that underlie retirement financial planning.

_____ 1. Do you understand why an SEP or a Keogh might be your best retirement plan alternative?

_____ 2. Do you understand the difference between a defined benefit plan and a defined contribution plan?

_____ 3. Do you understand the tax advantages of tax deferral and tax deductibility?

_____ 4. Are you aware that the enormous tax advantages of retirement investing can cause the after-tax returns to exceed the pretax returns offered in the financial markets?

_____ 5. Do you know what percentage of your income you should contribute each year to meet your retirement goal and whether your current savings are adequate?

_____ 6. Do you have a basic understanding of investment management alternatives?

Since retirement savings often represent the single most important financial resource of mature professionals, it is important that appropriate time be spent in assuring their efficient management. Statistics indicate a surprising percentage of people retire with disappointing financial resources. While this book has discussed a number of important topics, please don't underestimate the importance of the final topic: retirement.

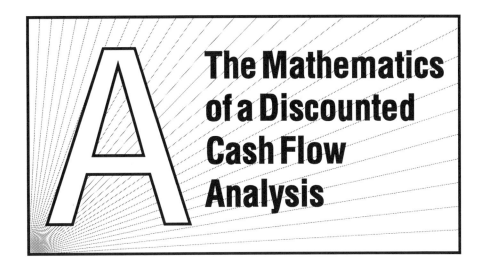

The Mathematics of a Discounted Cash Flow Analysis

The idea is to move each of the aggregate cash flows back to the current time period. This is accomplished by discounting each cash flow by the number of periods corresponding to the number of time periods before the cash flow will occur.

However, there is a time saving, shortcut method that we will demonstrate in this appendix. This will allow you to perform the final phase (discounting) in a quick and easy manner.

Figure A-1 focuses on the fifth column of a new four-year example. This will be used to demonstrate our shortcut for how the final column can be discounted, resulting in a final Bottom Line Result.

In a nutshell, the shortcut starts with the last period's value and moves upward, one period at a time, while discounting and summing in new values.

The shortcut method begins by entering the final year figure, in our example −$6,000, into a calculator. Next we discount the figure back from year four to year three and then add it to the figure for year three. The new sum is then discounted back for another year and summed into the figure from year two. The process is continued until the last figure (Period 0) has been summed into the total. Recall that a figure can be discounted for one year by dividing the figure by one plus the interest rate (expressed as a decimal).

If a cash flow is negative (as it usually will be in our analyses) then it should be subtracted. If it is positive, it should be added.

Let's do the method in detail using a discount rate of 12 percent. The method will alternate between summing and discounting from year four back to year zero. First, the −$6,000 final year figure is entered into the calculator and discounted for one year at

FIGURE A-1
EXAMPLE OF SHORTCUT METHOD

Time Period	(5) Total Cash Flow for Period
0	−1,600
1	+3,000
2	+1,800
3	+1,600
4	−6,000
Bottom Line Result	

12 percent by dividing the −$6,000 by 1.12. The result is −$5,357.14 rounded to the nearest cent. The keystrokes on a typical calculator would be:

−6000 ÷ 1.12 =

The year three value is summed in by keystroking:

+ 1600 =

Producing a new subtotal of −$3,757.14 (rounded). This new subtotal is again discounted to year two through division by one plus the interest rate (expressed as a decimal) by the following keystrokes:

÷1.12 =

The above keystrokes produce a new subtotal of −$3,354.59. The year two figure of $1,800 is summed to produce a new subtotal of −$1,554.59. The process continues, discounting to −$1,388.03 and then summing the year one figure to produce $1,611.97, discounting again to produce $1,439.26 and summing to produce the final result of −$160.74. Thus, this method allows the whole analysis to be collapsed into a single value that reflects today's dollars.

To speed up the process even further, you can try two shortcuts. First, most calculators will allow you to skip all of the equal signs. Second, store the quantity one plus the interest rate in a memory such that it can be retrieved by hitting the recall memory (e.g., RM) button. Using these shortcuts, all of the problem can be solved using only these keystrokes: [start by storing 1.12 into the memory and using RM to denote the memory recall button]

−6000 ÷ RM + 1600 ÷ RM + 1800 ÷ RM + 3000 ÷ RM − 1600 =

The final figure is the netted sum of all of the cash flows discounted for the time value of money.

There is a final note if your analysis uses time periods other than years, such as quarters. You can still use the above procedure except that the interest rate used should be based upon the length of the time period. Thus, a quarterly or monthly rate should be used. Annual rates can be turned into approximate periodic rates by dividing the annual rate by the number of time periods in a year (i.e., 4 for quarterly, 12 for monthly, and so forth). Thus instead of using 12 percent per year, you would use 3 percent per quarter or 1 percent per month.

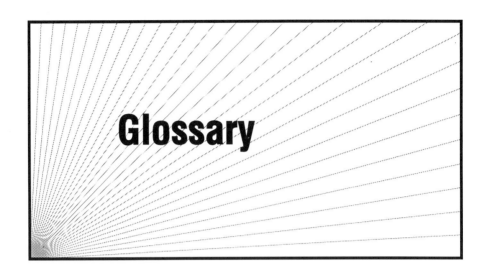

Glossary

401(k) A type of retirement plan in the form of a savings plan.

Accelerated Method of Depreciation A method of depreciation where a large portion of the asset is written off (converted to expense) in the early years of its life.

Accounting Journal An accounting record used to record individual financial transactions. Specific accounting journals exist for different types of transactions; see Cash Receipts Journal and Cash Disbursements Journal.

Accounting System A record keeping system that begins with the initial recording of a single financial transaction and ends with a summary of all financial activity for the operating period.

Accounts Payable Days Outstanding Number of days in the accounting period divided by accounts payable turnover. This ratio tells you on average how long it takes to pay your suppliers.

Accounts Payable Turnover The amount of credit purchases for the period divided by the accounts payable balance. This ratio tells you how many times you pay your suppliers in a given cycle.

Accounts Receivable Arise when you render services on credit with the promise by a patient to pay cash in the future.

Accounts Receivable Collection Period Number of days in the accounting period divided by accounts receivable turnover. This ratio tells you on average how long it takes to collect amounts due.

Accounts Receivable Turnover Services rendered on credit during the period divided by the accounts receivable balance. This ratio tells you how many times you collect your accounts receivable in a given cycle.

Accrued Pension Liability The amount owed to the pension plan that has not yet been deposited with the pension plan administrator.

Accumulated Depreciation The total amount of the depreciation recorded over the life of the asset.

ACRS (Accelerated Cost Recovery System) An accelerated depreciation method used for tax purposes.

Additional Contributed Capital See Additional Paid-In Capital.

Additional Paid-In Capital The contributed capital received at stock issuance in excess of the par or stated value of the common stock.

Adjusting Entry Additional periodic journal entries used to ensure that all relevant financial transactions are recorded in a given time period.

Administrative Expense Expense that results from the management (in contrast to the operation) of the practice.

Administrative Expense Percentage Total administrative expenses divided by professional fees earned.

Allowance for Bad Debts (This account appears only under an accrual basis.) An estimate of the amount of accounts receivable that the medical practice will be unable to collect; it reduces the value of accounts receivable.

Amortization The periodic allocation to expense of the dollars invested in intangibles, e.g., goodwill.

Asset Turnover Net sales divided by total assets.

Assets The financial resources owned, and available for use, by the medical practice.

Audit Evaluation by an independent third party, who objectively determines that the financial results reported by a business are reasonable.

Auditor's Opinion A statement by an independent third party as to the reasonableness of the financial information presented by a business.

Authorized Stock The number of shares a corporation can legally issue, consistent with the company's charter.

Balance Sheet Same as the Statement of Assets, Liabilities and Equity. This financial statement discloses information on the practice's financial position at a specific point in time. This statement lists the financial resources (assets), the financial obligations (liabilities), and ownership rights (equity) within the practice.

Bank Reconciliation (Bank Reconcilement) A process used to identify differences between the cash balance shown in the general ledger cash account and the cash balance reported on a bank statement.

Benefit Obligation The liability for future payments associated with a pension plan.

Bonding The purchase of an insurance policy to protect against employee theft.

Book Depreciation Depreciation recorded in the financial accounting records. Methods of book depreciation are: straight line, units of production, sum of the year's digits, and double declining balance.

Book Value Cost of an asset less its accumulated depreciation.

Capital Lease Leasing arrangement where the lessee seeks a long-term commitment to use the asset; it is similar to purchasing an asset.

Capital Structure Ratios Ratios which identify the creditor (debt) versus ownership (equity) positions within a business. Common capital structure ratios are: Current Debt to Equity, Long-Term Debt to Equity, Debt to Equity, and Times Interest Earned.

Cash Basis The accounting method which records financial transactions at the time cash is received or paid.

Cash Disbursements Journal The accounting record used to show all cash outlays of the practice.

Cash Equivalents Short-term highly liquid investments with original maturities of less than three months.

Cash Ratio Cash and cash-type assets divided by outstanding current liabilities.

Cash Receipts Journal The accounting record used to show all cash inflows to the practice.

Closing Entries Journal entries which result in a zero balance in all revenue and expense accounts. These entries are recorded only at the end of an accounting period.

Common Stock A share of stock which indicates ownership in a corporation.

Common-Size Statements Financial statements which reduce each element to a common denominator.

Comparative Data A practice's financial data from prior years as well as relevant industry data; they are often used in financial statement analysis.

Compilation Accounting services performed by an accountant not employed by the medical practice. These services are limited to preparing financial statements based on information recorded by the medical practice.

Contingencies Potential liabilities of a business.

Contingent Liabilities See Contingencies.

Contributed Capital Ownership interest in a corporation resulting from a stock issue.

Contribution Carry-Forward A tax benefit for which contributions made in excess of IRS regulations can be carried forward to future periods.

Contributory Pension Plan A pension plan in which the employee makes a contribution (payment).

Corporation A distinct legal entity with rights and liabilities separate from those of the shareholders.

Current Assets Financial resources in cash form or those which can be converted to cash within one year, or the operating cycle, whichever is longer.

Current Debt to Equity Ratio Current liabilities divided by stockholder's equity.

Current Liabilities Debts which mature within one year, or the operating cycle, whichever is longer.

Current Ratio Current assets divided by current liabilities.

Debt/Equity Ratio Total debt divided by total stockholder's equity.

Debt and Equity Mix The combination of debt and equity used to finance a business.

Debt and Equity Structure The percentage of assets supported by debt, versus that which is supported by equity.

Deferred Taxes A long-term liability that represents a temporary postponement of the federal tax obligation to a period exceeding one year from the date of the financial statements.

Defined Benefit Plan A pension plan sponsored by the employer where a specific, defined retirement benefit is to be paid to an employee.

Defined Contribution Plan A pension plan sponsored by the employer whereby the employer commits a predetermined amount each accounting period to the pension plan.

Depreciation Expense The charge against current period income to reflect the use of buildings and equipment during that time period.

Direct Costs Costs that are clearly and directly associated with rendering services.

Disclosure Notes See Footnote Disclosure.

Discount Rate The interest rate used to adjust a future cash flow to its present value.

Discounting The process of adjusting for the time value of money.

Double Entry Bookkeeping System Entering every financial transaction in the accounting system as two components: cash received (paid) and source (destination) of cash.

Extraordinary Gain or Loss Transactions that are both unusual in nature and infrequent in occurrence.

Financial Results A report summarizing the financial transactions over a period of time.

Financial Statement Analysis A logical and systematic method of examining, summarizing, and interpreting financial statement data.

Financial Statements The standard mechanism used to summarize the financial results of a company's business operations.

Financing Activity A classification on the Statement of Cash Flows. It describes transactions that involve obtaining or repaying debt or obtaining or repurchasing stock.

Fixed Assets The property and equipment of a medical practice.

Fixed Costs Costs which do not vary with changes in the level (volume) of operations.

Fixed Income Investments Securities that offer relatively fixed or predetermined rates of return.

Footnote Disclosures Supplemental financial information in narrative form that provides support for, or details of, the numbers reported in the financial statements.

Funding Policy The method used to accumulate pension plan assets.

General Ledger The master accounting record containing all of the accounts used in the accounting system. It is the source of the numerical information reported in the financial statements.

General Partnership A form of business organization which brings two or more persons together as co-owners.

Goodwill The intangible asset that arises when the acquisition cost of a practice is in excess of the book value of its net assets.

Incidental Transactions The revenues, expenses, gains, or losses earned or incurred outside of a medical practice's normal operating activity.

Income before Tax Percentage Income before taxes divided by total professional fees earned.

Income from Operations Percentage Income from operations divided by total professional fees earned.

Income Tax Basis The recording of revenues and expenses in the same manner as they are reported on a tax return.

Indirect Costs Costs that are incidental or not related to the direct function of treating patients.

Individual Retirement Account (IRA) A type of retirement plan used by any individual who receives compensation during a year.

Intangibles An asset, such as goodwill, that does not have physical form or substance.

Internal Controls Policies and procedures used to ensure that business assets are used and accounted for in a manner consistent with management's intent.

Investing Activity A classification on the Statement of Cash Flows which involves transactions affecting the productive resources of a medical practice.

Invoice Payment Terms Number of days allowed before payment of the invoice to the supplier is required.

IRA See Individual Retirement Account.

Issued Stock The shares of stock initially sold to the associates of the medical practice.

Journal Entry The vehicle used to record a financial transaction in the accounting system.

Keogh A type of retirement plan for a sole proprietor or partnership used for the exclusive benefit of the employees.

Law of Agency Legal principle which states that if a person is acting as your agent, you may be held responsible for his or her actions.

Lease An arrangement which allows one person or organization to use an asset while another person or organization owns the asset.

Legal Capital Common stock par value recorded at issuance.

Lessee One who "rents" the asset in the leasing arrangement.

Lessor One who originally owns the asset in the leasing arrangement.

Liabilities The financial obligations (debt) of a business incurred to support and maintain the business operations.

Limited Liability Company (LLC) A form of business organization under which participants can be involved in the management of the business without subjecting themselves to personal liability.

Limited Partnership A form of business organization which brings two or more persons together as co-owners and some protection against personal liability is obtained.

Liquidity The cash position of a company; indicates the ability to use current assets to pay off current liabilities on a dollar for dollar basis.

Liquidity Ratios Ratios measuring the cash position of a company; usually an indication of a company's ability to pay short-term debt obligations on a timely basis.

Long-Term Debt Debt due after one year.

Long-Term Debt to Equity Ratio Long term debt divided by stockholder's equity.

Long-Term Liabilities See Long-Term Debt.

MACRS (Modified Accelerated Cost Recovery System) An accelerated depreciation method used for tax purposes under current tax law.

Management The operating and financial officers of the practice; they are responsible for the financial statement information.

Marginal Cost The next dollar spent to generate one additional dollar in professional fees.

Market Value Current exchange price as of the date of the financial statement.

Matching Principle The accounting principle which requires the offset of expenses against the revenue reported in an accounting period.

Medical Supplies Expense Expense for supplies consumed when you render medical services.

Minimum Future Lease Payments Payment that the lessee is required to make by contract to the lessor; includes any penalty for not renewing the lease.

Mutual Fund A corporation that pools funds from many investors and manages the funds with specific investment objectives.

Net Income The net of revenues, expenses, gains, and losses, over a specified period of time.

Net Income Percentage Net income divided by total professional fees earned.

Net Working Capital Current assets minus current liabilities.

No-Par Stock Stock which does not assign par or stated value.

Noncontributory Pension Plan A pension plan where contributions are made by the employer rather than the employee.

Nonrepetitive Transactions Those transactions that are unusual and infrequent in nature; they are often transactions incidental to the primary purpose of a medical practice.

Note Disclosure See Footnote Disclosures.

Notes to the Financial Statements See Footnote Disclosures.

Off–Balance Sheet Financing Can exist in the form of a lease agreement, i.e., not reporting the existing lease liability on the Statement of Assets, Liabilities and Equity because it is classified as an operating lease.

Operating Activity A classification on the Statement of Cash Flows which describes cash flows resulting from normal business operations.

Operating Expense Percentage Total operating expense divided by total professional fees earned.

Operating Lease A lease with no transfer of ownership interest; annual rent commitments are recorded as rental expense in the current period as they occur.

Operating Loss Carry-Forward A tax benefit which allows losses in a current period to offset taxable income in a subsequent period.

Outstanding Stock Shares of stock that have been issued and are still held by a shareholder.

Paid in Excess of Par The amount received at issuance in excess of the par or stated value of the common stock.

Partnership See General Partnership and/or Limited Partnership.

Par Value The amount assigned to a particular stock by the corporation within the limits of the incorporating state.

Payroll Tax Expense Payroll taxes paid by the practice for each employee; it does not included payroll taxes withheld from employees' paychecks.

Pension Benefit Guarantee Corporation (PBGC) A government agency which insures pension benefit plans, monitors existing funds, and administers plans for bankrupt companies.

Pension Obligation A company's commitment during the retirement years of their employees. It is based on the services rendered by employees in earlier years.

Pension Plan Assets The resources owned by a pension plan.

Principal The cash you spend to repay a loan and reduce your indebtedness.

Professional Corporation (PC) A form of business organization where substantially all of the stock must be owned directly by the employees who perform(ed) services to the corporation.

Profit The difference between revenues and expenses when revenues are in excess of expenses.

Profit and Loss Statement See Statement of Income.

Quick Ratio Cash, short-term investments, and receivables divided by current liabilities.

Ratio Analysis A significant component of financial statement analysis. Ratio analysis summarizes financial statement relationships among the financial statement elements.

Receivables A short-term asset resulting from services rendered on credit; it represents a patient's balance due to the practice.

Return on Assets (ROA) Net income divided by total assets.

Review An accounting service provided by an accountant not employed by the practice. This service includes preparation of the financial statements from the accounting records of the medical practice and other limited procedures, such as inquiry of employees.

Risk Assessment An assimilation of data which simplifies the assigning of priorities to apparent risk factors.

"S" Corporation A form of business organization which allows shareholders to pay taxes at individual tax rates.

Section 179 Carry-Forward A tax benefit which arises when a business is not able to use all of the section 179 benefits allowed by IRS code in a given time period.

Semivariable Costs "Step costs" which are fixed up to a certain level of operations; upon reaching a predetermined level, these costs become variable.

Shareholders' Equity The ownership interest of an organization; it is the residual amount after liabilities are subtracted from assets.

Short-Term Debt Those debts which mature within one year or the operating cycle whichever is longer.

Short-Term Liabilities See Short-Term Debt.

Simplified Employee Pension (SEP) A pension plan which allows you to make contributions for both owners and employees based on compensation.

Sole Proprietorship A form of business organization under which the owner and the business are not considered separate legal entities.

Stated Value The value assigned to any stock. For accounting purposes, this is the same as par value.

Statement of Cash Flows A financial statement which summarizes the current period business activities on a cash basis.

Statement of Changes in Shareholders' Equity A financial statement which identifies the balance of, and the changes in, specific owner's equity accounts listed on the Statement of Assets, Liabilities and Equity.

Statement of Earnings See Statement of Income.

Statement of Income A report of a company's revenues, expenses, gains, and losses that are the result of operating and nonoperating activities over a specific period of time.

Statement of Income and Retained Earnings A statement which combines the Statement of Income and the Statement of Retained Earnings.

Statement of Revenue and Expenses See Income Statement.

Statement of Stockholders' Equity See Statement of Changes in Shareholders' Equity.

Stockholders' Equity See Shareholders' Equity.

Straight-Line Depreciation A uniform write-off of dollars over the life of buildings or equipment.

Summary of Significant Accounting Policies The first footnote disclosure with the financial statements; this footnote identifies the financial processes used in the practice to record accounting information and prepare financial reports.

Supplemental Schedule A form of note disclosure that provides detailed support for the numerical information presented in total in the financial statements.

Tax Deferral The delay of the payment of taxes from one year to a later year.

Tax Depreciation Depreciation recorded for tax purposes.

Treasury Stock Shares of stock that have been issued but have been reacquired by the practice and are no longer owned by an associate.

Trend Analysis An analysis which facilitates the identification and understanding of specific trends.

Trial Balance Part of a verification phase in the accounting cycle: it lists all general ledger accounts and their respective credit or debit balances.

Variable Costs Costs which change directly with changes in the level (volume) of operations.

Working Capital Current assets less current liabilities.

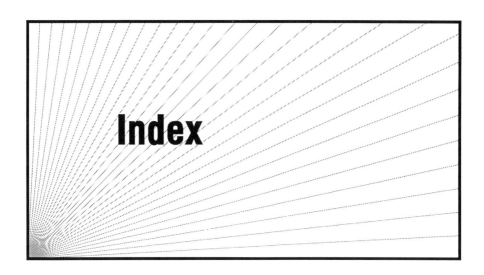

Index

interest to debts, 65
internal controls, 130*f*
  importance of, 122-25, 129-31, 141-42
  procedures for, 125-31, 139-42
    cash disbursements, 133*f,* 134-35,
      137*f,* 138
    cash receipts, 131-35, 136*f*
    payroll, 138-39
Internal Revenue Service (IRS). *See also*
    taxes, *individual forms of*
  on basis of reporting, 46
  on depreciation, 87, 101, 108, 116
  on eligible employees, 113
  on estimated taxes, 62
  on LLC determination, 30
  on professional corporations, 29
  on rental payments, 115
  on retirement plans, 166
  on "S" corporations, 27
inventory, 47-48, 63, 85
investment. *See also* retirement investing;
    shareholders' equity, *individual com-
    ponents of*
  activities of, 42, 80, 95-96, 98
  in another practice, 64
  in assets, 96
  in equities, 181-82
  fees of, 183-84
  fixed income, 181-84
  horizon of, 181
  rate of return, 173*f*
  in securities, 61, 95
  in ventures, 114
IRA (Individual Retirement Arrangements),
    167
IRS. *See* Internal Revenue Service (IRS)
journals, accounting. *See* accounting sys-
    tem, *individual journals of*

K–L

Keogh retirement plan, 167

labor costs, 90
land as asset, 63
Law of Agency, 20
leasehold improvements, 63-64
leasing, 143-44
  versus buying, 163. *See also* cost/benefit
    analysis
  capital leases, 145, 163
  operating leases, 144-45
  sales and leasebacks, 145

tax benefits of, 148-50. *See also* deprecia-
    tion, tax benefits of
  types of leases, 114-15, 163
liabilities, 5, 11-12, 58. *See also* expenses;
    Statement of Assets, Liabilities and
    Equity
  accrued pension, 65
  arrangement of, 60
  classifying, 69
  current, 64
  income tax payable, 66
  line of credit, 65-66
  long-term, 64, 66
  maturity of, 76
  mortgage payable, current portion of, 66
  notes payable, 64-66
  order of arrangement, 76
  payroll taxes withheld, 65-66
  pension expense, 112
  valuation of, 61
liability. *See* business organization, *individ-
    ual forms of*
liability risks, protection from, 145
Limited Liability Company. *See* business or-
    ganization, Limited Liability Company
limited liability concept, 24
limited partnership. *See* business organiza-
    tion, limited partnership
liquidity, 71-73, 76
LLC. *See* business organization, Limited Li-
    ability Company
loans, 65-66
loss, 39, 41, 78, 116

M–N

MACRS (Modified Accelerated Cost Recov-
    ery System), 87, 108
maintenance and repair expenditures, 109
malpractice, 22-23
managed care organizations, 21
marginal cost, 91
marginal revenue, 91
marketable securities, 61
materials cost, 90
maturity of liabilities, 76
Modified Accelerated Cost Recovery System
    (MACRS), 87, 108
modified cash basis of accounting, 17, 46-
    49, 49*f*
money, present value of, 156
money purchase plans, 167
mortgages, 61, 66

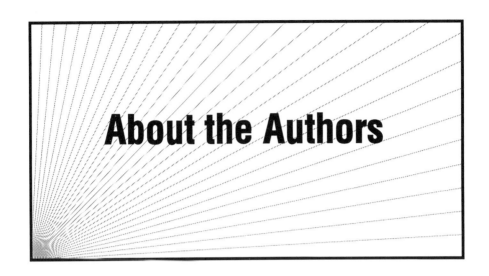

About the Authors

Rose Marie L. Bukics

Rose Marie L. Bukics is currently a professor and the Chair of the Department of Economics and Business at LaFayette College. She joined LaFayette College in 1980 after serving as an auditor for the "Big Eight" firm of Deloitte, Haskins and Sells. Bukics graduated summa cum laude from the University of Scranton and received her MBA from Lehigh University. A certified public accountant in the state of Pennsylvania, Bukics has previously written and edited four books about financial management and is a member of the American Institute of Certified Public Accountants, the Pennsylvania Institute of Certified Public Accountants, and the American Accounting Association.

Donald R. Chambers

Donald R. Chambers currently serves as the Walter E. Hanson/KPMG Peat Marwick Professor of Finance at LaFayette College where he teaches corporate finance and investments and serves as the advisor to the Investments Club. He received his Ph.D. from the University of North Carolina at Chapel Hill in 1981.

Dr. Chambers has published over twenty articles in finance journals and in 1994 he published a textbook entitled *Modern Corporate Finance: Theory and Practice.* Dr. Chambers frequently serves as a consultant to the public and private sectors.